THE UNIVE
WINCH~~ESTER~~

Disability, Culture and Identity

PEARSON

Education

We work with leading authors to develop the strongest educational materials in social studies, bringing cutting-edge thinking and best learning practice to a global market.

Under a range of well-known imprints, including Prentice Hall, we craft high quality print and electronic publications which help readers to understand and apply their content, whether studying or at work.

To find out more about the complete range of our publishing, please visit us on the World Wide Web at: www.pearsoneduc.com

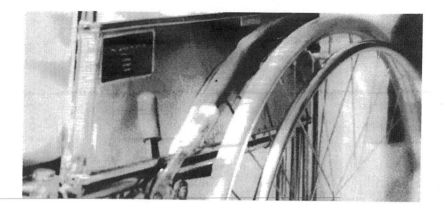

Disability, Culture and Identity

Sheila Riddell
Nick Watson

Harlow, England • London • New York • Boston • San Francisco • Toronto • Sydney • Singapore • Hong Kong
Tokyo • Seoul • Taipei • New Delhi • Cape Town • Madrid • Mexico City • Amsterdam • Munich • Paris • Milan

Pearson Education Limited
Edinburgh Gate
Harlow
Essex CM20 2JE
United Kingdom

and Associated Companies throughout the world

Visit us on the World Wide Web at:
www.pearsoneduc.com

First published 2003
© Pearson Education Limited 2003

ISBN 0 130 89440 0

British Library Cataloguing-in-Publication Data
A catalogue record for this book is available from the British Library

Transferred to digital print on demand, 2007

Typeset in 10/12.5 pt Book Antiqua by 35
Produced by Pearson Education Malaysia Sdn Bhd,
Printed and bound by CPI Antony Rowe, Eastbourne

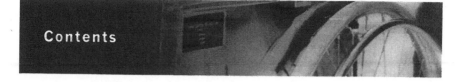

Contents

CHAPTER ONE

Disability, Culture and Identity: Introduction   1

Sheila Riddell and Nick Watson

CHAPTER TWO

A culture of participation?   19

E. Kay M. Tisdall

CHAPTER THREE

CHAPTER FOUR

CHAPTER FIVE

CHAPTER SIX

Deafness/Disability – problematising notions of identity, culture and structure

Mairian Scott-Hill

CHAPTER SEVEN

Against a politics of victimisation: disability culture and self-advocates with learning difficulties

Danny Goodley

CHAPTER EIGHT

Now I Know Why Disability Art is Drowning in the River Lethe (with thanks to Pierre Bourdieu)   131

Paul Anthony Darke

CHAPTER NINE

Mainstreaming disability on Radio 4   143

Brian Sweeney and Sheila Riddell

CHAPTER TEN

Disability and ethnicity: how young Asian disabled people make sense of their lives   161

Karl Atkin and Yasmin Hussain

CHAPTER ELEVEN

Can multiculturalism encompass disability?   180

Andrew Jakubowicz and Helen Meekosha

Sheila Riddell
Strathclyde Centre for Disability Research
University of Glasgow

Nick Watson
Department of Nursing Studies
University of Edinburgh

Mark Priestley
Disability Research Unit
University of Leeds

Mairian Scott-Hill
School of Education
Kings College London

Kay Tisdall
Children in Scotland
Edinburgh

Brian Sweeney
Strathclyde Centre for Disability Research
University of Glasgow

Iain Ferguson
Department of Applied Social Studies
University of Stirling

Danny Goodley
Department of Education
University of Sheffield

Paul Anthony Darke
Outside Centre Limited
www.outside-centre.com

Karl Atkin
Centre for Research in Primary Care
Nuffield Institute for Health
University of Leeds

Yasmin Hussain
Department of Social Policy
University of Leeds

Andrew Jakubowicz
Department of Journalism, Writing and Social Inquiry
University of Technology, Sydney

Helen Meekosha
School of Social Work
University of New South Wales

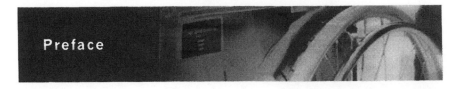

Preface

Much has been written about the ways in which economic inequalities shape people's life chances in capitalist societies. Whilst recognising the fundamental importance of access to physical resources, this book reflects the view that access to social and cultural capital may be just as important as access to financial resources in structuring both life chances and emotions. The disability movement has drawn attention to the economic and cultural oppression experienced by disabled people. This book focuses on the ways in which this oppression varies in relation to a range of social factors such as social class, 'race' and gender and the nature of an individual's impairment. It also considers the ways in which art and the media are implicated in cultural denial, and the various resistances which are employed. We hope that it will contribute to ongoing debates in relation to social theories of disability.

We would like to thank all those who have been involved in the ongoing ESRC Disability Studies seminars which inspired this book. The seminars were initially run by Len Barton, subsequently by Nick Watson and Sheila Riddell and, at the time of writing, by Colin Barnes. We believe that the seminars have been immensely valuable in contributing to the growing field of disability studies, and we would like to thank the ESRC for support over the past decade.

This book inevitably reflects a particular perspective on the field of disability, culture and identity. We see it not as 'the last word', but as a contribution to a dynamic and evolving area which will undoubtedly look very different ten years down the line.

Sheila Riddell
Nick Watson
7 January 2003

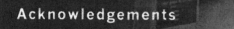

Acknowledgements

Every book is a joint project between many people, and in this spirit we would like to thank our colleagues at Edinburgh and Glasgow Universities and all the participants in the ESRC-funded seminar series *Disability and the Restructuring of Welfare* which took place between 1997 and 2000. The Disability Studies seminar series, which was launched by Professor Len Barton in 1996 and is being continued by Professor Colin Barnes, has acted as an important catalyst in the development of disability studies scholarship in the UK and we wish it a long and evolving life.

Many thanks to Jean McPartland for her excellent administrative support in organising the seminars and in the preparation of the manuscript.

On a personal note, Nick would like to thank Mandy, and Sheila would like to thank Ken, Annie and Bella for their love and support.

CHAPTER 1

Disability, Culture and Identity: Introduction

Sheila Riddell and Nick Watson

Introduction

The aim of this book is to explore disability and impairment through the lens of culture. The socially dominant culture shapes the way in which disability and impairment are viewed, and has contributed to the oppression of disabled people. At the same time disabled people have forged their own cultures as acts of resistance. Culture, therefore, is both a source of oppression and of liberation for disabled people, and is therefore central to the politics of disability. Acknowledging the importance of culture in shaping social structures is seen by some in the disability movement as potentially dangerous or threatening, in that it may throw up unwanted complexities which distract attention away from the political struggle against oppression. However, in producing this book we do not feel that we have launched into a self-indulgent and diversionary 'cultural turn'. Rather, we seek to contribute to the vibrancy of the disability movement and disability studies by recognising the centrality of culture in shaping social relationships. By unearthing and pursuing some of the tensions and debates between social modellists and cultural theorists, we believe that the field of disability studies will be enriched and the disability movement in general will become more sensitive to difference, ultimately contributing to its resilience and effectiveness.

Throughout this book, we explore disability and culture from a sociological standpoint. Sociology, as Brian Turner and Chris Rojeck (2001) have recently argued, starts with an investigation of everyday life and the relationships and conditions that shape it, which are themselves imbued with elements of culture. As Mike Oliver and colleagues (in press) have noted, sociology has a crucial role to play in disability studies because of its emphasis on issues of equality, justice and power. We hope that this book illustrates the political relevance, rather than sterility, of studying disability and culture from a sociological perspective.

In contrast with earlier writing which focused on disability as social and economic oppression, disabled people have recently come to see cultural revaluation as central to their political struggle. Writers such as Anne Karpf (1988), Tom Shakespeare (1994), David Hevey (1992) Martin Norden (1994) and Lois Keith (2000) have sought to show how images of disabled people are used to in the media and in literature. They point to the media fondness for cure stories; the role of charity appeals; the invisibility of disabled people on television; the stereotyped portrayal of disabled characters in screen drama; the under-employment of disabled people in broadcasting; the representation of disabled people as flawed or damaged. As noted above, this emphasis on representation of disabled people still causes concern for some within the disabled people's movement (Barnes and Mercer 2001). The criticism is that if disability studies abandons an agenda of redistribution and equality in favour of an emphasis on difference and diversity it could potentially lead to an uncritical acceptance of structural inequality as an expression of cultural difference. Some have argued that the politics of cultural recognition and the politics of economic redistribution may be complementary rather than at odds with each other. A central theme of this book is to consider, with regard to disability, whether economic and cultural struggles are mutually supportive or contradictory.

The social model of disability and culture

In order to understand the origins of the tensions between disability studies and cultural studies, we need to look at the early writing of the disability movement. As Thomas (1999) has noted, the social model of disability was generated as a result of the efforts of disability activists to identify some fundamental principles to inform their actions. The Union of Physically Impaired Against Segregation (UPIAS) produced a document in 1976 entitled *Fundamental Principles of Disability*. This document set out the following definitions of impairment and disability:

> *Impairment:* 'lacking all or part of a limb, or having a defective limb, organ or mechanism of the body.'

> *Disability*: 'the disadvantage or restriction of activity caused by a contemporary social organisation which takes no or little account of people who have physical impairments and thus excludes them from the mainstream of social activities.'   (reprinted in Oliver 1996, p. 22)

This socio-political definition of disability was subsequently broadened to accommodate people with a range of impairments, including those with physical and sensory impairments, learning difficulties and mental health problems (Barnes 1996). It has been suggested that early writers within the field of disability studies had very little to say about the personal experience of disability, its cultural elements and the impact these had on individual identities (Thomas 1999; Shakespeare 1996; Shakespeare *et al.* 1996). Looking back at Mike Oliver's seminal book *The Politics of Disablement* (Oliver 1990), it is evident that culture was not ignored, but it was construed in a relatively uncomplicated way. According to Oliver, the oppression of disabled people was at root economic, but ideologies about disabled people played a part in maintaining existing inequalities. Thus in art and literature, disabled people were presented as either super-heroes, villains or tragic individuals, but never as ordinary people trying to carve out meaningful lives, like everybody else. The remedy for this cultural oppression was for disabled people to challenge these ideologies, forging new identities which challenged outworn stereotypes. The disability arts movement features in Oliver's later writing (Oliver 1996; Campbell and Oliver 1996), its work construed as acts of political resistance. *The Politics of Disablement*, however, contains a crushing attack on medical and psychological approaches to disability which emphasise the need for the disabled individual to adjust to the conditions of impairment. Since there is no theoretical or empirical grounding for such an approach, Oliver concluded that it must be rooted in the dominant cultural paradigm of disability as personal tragedy:

> ... professionals are clearly influenced by cultural images and ideological constructions of disability as an individual, medical and tragic problem. The issue of adjustment, therefore, became the focus for professional intervention and reinforced these very images and constructions by rooting them in practice.   (Oliver 1990, p. 64)

Reluctance to draw on cultural studies, with its emphasis on the negotiation of multiple and shifting identities, may well stem from ongoing suspicion of traditional medical and psychological approaches which pathologise disabled individuals.

Proponents of the social model of disability, therefore, argued that disabled people should concentrate on developing a shared cultural politics which focused on the material causes of oppression. Reflection on the individual meaning of disability was seen as potentially dangerous since it might fragment, rather than unite, the movement. However, criticisms of the social model of disability have been expressed by those who argue the case for investigating the complexity of disability, culture and identity. Writers like Crow (1996), for example, maintained that the personal experience of impairment had been downplayed because acknowledging individual pain and oppression did not necessarily accord with the view that disability was entirely a product of social barriers. Comparing the struggles for equality in the areas of 'race', gender and disability, she noted:

> There is nothing inherently unpleasant or difficult about other people's embodiment: sexuality, sex or colour are neutral facts. In contrast, our experience of impairment means our experiences of our bodies can be unpleasant or difficult. This does not mean our campaigns against disability are any less vital than those against heterosexism, sexism or racism; it does mean that for many disabled people personal struggle related to impairment will remain even when disabling barriers no longer exist.   (Crow 1996, p. 58)

Similarly, Shakespeare (1996) argued for the importance of exploring disability and sexuality in order to forge links between the personal and the political domains:

> In general, with the exception of the feminist literature on disabled women, there has been little emphasis in disability studies on the realm of identity, personal experience and private life. For us, the personal is political and, while we understood that the priority had been to explore structural relations and social barriers in the public spheres of life, we felt it was high time to redress the balance.   (Shakespeare 1996, p. 179)

Challenges to the social model of disability have also come from those who argue that disability studies has paid insufficient attention to the cultural politics of 'race', gender and age (see, for example, chapters

in this book by Atkin *et al.*, Jakubowicz and Meekosha, and Priestley).
Thomas (1999) suggests that such challenges have certainly put the
social model of disability, as the rallying point for the movement, under
strain. Yet the overall impact of such debates has been to enrich the
emerging field of disability studies.

What is culture?

Culture, as a concept, is broad and diffuse and it is important to establish some of the things we might mean by the word itself. Cultural
Studies is an immensely popular area of study, having its roots in the
work of writers such as Raymond Williams and Richard Hoggart, who,
influenced by their working class origins, wished to understand the relationship between the life practices and beliefs of working class people
and the dominant culture of the middle class. Writing in the 1950s, these
writers maintained that culture and society could not be separated, and
that people's family, social, and recreational lives, the clothes they wore
and the newspapers they read, were imbued with political significance. Culture, as Williams (1976/1988, p. 87) has observed, is one of the
most complicated words in the English language. It is also one of the
key concepts in modern social knowledge. In its early usage it described
the process of tending crops or animals. In the sixteenth century the
concept was extended to include culture as the process of human
development. In the late eighteenth and early nineteenth century the
concept of culture as a noun emerged. This understanding places culture, or cultures, as a descriptor of the 'configuration or generalisation'
of a group of people (Williams 1981, p. 10). The concept served to
describe the way of life of particular groups, peoples or eras. Later, with
the publication of Matthew Arnold's *Culture and Anarchy*, the word
came to be associated with the arts, specifically the 'high arts' such
as classical music, painting, sculpture, theatre and certain types of film.
At the end of the nineteenth century what Williams termed the *social*
definition of culture emerged.

The social definition of culture emphasises culture as a 'signifying
system' as a packet of signs, symbols, tools and beliefs. Through this
system 'a social order is communicated, reproduced, experienced and
explored' (Williams 1981, p. 13). This idea originated in the work of the
anthropologist Franz Boas, the sociologist Emile Durkheim and the
linguist Ferdinand de Saussure (Friedman 1994). This notion of culture has dominated much writing on culture throughout the twentieth
century.

> A culture has two aspects: the known meanings and directions, which its members are trained to; the new observations and meanings, which are offered and tested. These are the ordinary processes of human societies and human minds, and we see through them the nature of a culture: that it is always both traditional and creative; that it is both the most ordinary common meanings and the finest common meanings. We use the word culture in these two senses: to mean a whole way of life – the common meanings; to mean the arts and learning – the special processes of discovery and creative effort.   (Williams 1989, p. 4)

Culture and disability

Disability is, as writers such as Oliver (1990, 1996), Colin Barnes *et al.* (2000) and John Swain *et al.* (1994) point out, linked to notions of inequality of power and human interdependence. While the emphasis in disability studies has, until recently, tended to explore disablement through economic rather than cultural processes, the latter have always been part of the equation. So, for example, Oliver (1990), linked the oppression of disabled people to the material changes associated with capitalist development. However, he also identified ideological changes which were needed to challenge oppression. Disability is not, according to Oliver, 'defined or culturally produced solely in terms of its relationship to the mode of production' (1990, p. 22). He argues that disability is culturally produced through the relationship between the mode of production and the central values of society. Capitalist society has resulted in an ideology of individualism, which, coupled with medicalisation and the development of rehabilitation, brought about profound changes in the way that people with impairments are seen and treated. Oliver suggests that the ideologies of both individualism and medicalisation affect the individual experience of disability. In other words, the experience of disability is 'structured by the discursive practices which stem from these ideologies' (p. 58). Thus, what Oliver terms a 'hegemony of disability' (p. 44) emerges. By employing the Gramscian concept of hegemony, Oliver argues that these ideologies have become dominant and are part of the common sense view of disability as a 'personal tragedy'.

Oliver asserts the existence of a set of beliefs in British society which give coherence to this hegemony of disability. Norms are set and these norms are used to oppress disabled people:

The hegemony that defines disability in capitalist society is constituted by the organic ideology of individualism, the arbitrary ideologies of medicalisation underpinning medical intervention and personal tragedy theory underpinning much social policy. Incorporated also are ideologies related to concepts of normality, able-bodiedness and able-mindedness.

(1990, p. 44)

This assumption of the presence of a common sense view of disability, that of disability as tragedy, is important not just for Oliver's theorising, but, as discussed below, for many other writers on disability. This creates what Schutz (1970, pp. 72–76) would term a 'natural attitude' for people in their ordinary social existence. In Oliver's analysis, culture acts very much as structure, popular consciousness is manipulated by the medical profession and others who serve their own interests in presenting disabled people as tragic victims. That is, 'ordinary' people are one-dimensional and lack the critical capacity to challenge the dominant powers in society. This thesis is open to challenge (Abercrombie *et al.* 1980). In the writings of, for example, European sociologists such as Pierre Bourdieu (1986), culture is seen as the site of power struggles between different social groups. Bourdieu, developing the notion of 'habitus', suggested that the acquisition and transmission of social and cultural capital were powerful mechanisms for the reproduction of social inequality. Paul Willis, writing about a group of working class lads, explored the way in which they celebrated working class macho culture, which was for them a source of both power and oppression. A common thread in these writings was that, despite the expression of power relationships within and between cultures, sub-cultures were able to challenge and undermine the dominant culture. In relation to disability, there is a need first of all to consider whether it is possible to identify one, or several, cultures of disability and secondly, how these cultures relate to dominant social beliefs and values.

Shakespeare (1994) has criticised the social model for its failure to include culture fully in its analysis of disability and disablement. He notes the paucity of writings from social model theorists on cultural imagery, arguing that this stems from the neglect of impairment: 'If the social model analysis seeks to ignore, rather than explore, the individual experiences of impairment (be it blindness, short stature or whatever), then it is unsurprising that it should also gloss over cultural representation of impairment, because to do otherwise would be to potentially undermine the argument' (pp. 283–284). Drawing on the writings of Simone de Beauvoir, Victor Turner and Mary Douglas, he examines the cultural representation of disabled people in terms of otherness, ideology, anomaly and liminality. His work, alongside that of Hevey (1992), Darke (1998), Davis (1995) and the edited collection of Ingstad and Whyte (1995), explores how contemporary cultural representations of impairment generate disabling representations of the impaired body. These disabling images are every bit as oppressive as environmental or other material barriers. Shakespeare argues that such imagery promotes a fear of impairment:

> People project their fear of death, their unease at their physicality and mortality, onto disabled people, who represent all these different aspects of human existence. Disabled people are scapegoats. It is not just that disabled people are different, expensive, inconvenient or odd; it is that they represent a threat – either as Douglas suggests to order, or, to the self-conception of western beings – who, since the Enlightenment, have tried to view themselves as perfectible, as all knowing, as God like.
>
> (1994, p. 298)

This analysis is useful, in that cultural constructions of and about the body can sustain particular views and social relations (Scheper-Hughes and Lock 1987). For example, Needham (in Scheper-Hughes and Lock 1987), points out that the symbolic representation of the left as inferior, dark and dirty and the right as superior, light and dominant, is used to justify particular social values and social arrangements. However, there is a danger that Shakespeare's work could be used to suggest that such feelings are in some way essential to the experiences of impairment. By his failure to examine the origins of such cultural representations, his work runs the risk of reifying the view of disabled people as other, as found in the work of Pinder (1995, 1996).

Scheper-Hughes and Lock (1987) provide a useful corrective to this. They argue that as society has become increasingly 'healthist' and body-conscious, so the politically correct body has become lean, strong and physically fit (p. 25). Impairment and ill-health are no longer seen to arise as a consequence of bad luck or misfortune, but of an individual's failure to live right, eat well, exercise and so on. This individualisation of health can lead to stigmatisation of any who do not conform to the professionally determined 'norms'. Similarly, Robert Crawford argues that health has become '. . . an important symbolic domain for creating and recreating the self' (1994, p. 1356) and that the concept of health is central to modern identity. In a similar vein to that of Shakespeare, he further goes on to suggest that 'The "healthy self" is sustained in part through the creation of "unhealthy others", who are imagined as embodying all the properties falling outside this health signified self' (p. 1358).

Disability studies has, in the main, tended to react to, rather than provide new paradigms in, the fields of sociology connected to culture and cultural studies. So, for example, much of the writing emerging from disability studies on the sociology of the body has tended to downplay the importance of the body and the embodied nature of being (see for example Oliver 1996). Similarly disability studies has tended to promulgate the notion of the universal collective subject. This is in contrast to feminism, which under the influence of writers such as Judith Butler (1990), Diane Fuss (1989) and Nancy Fraser and Linda Nicholson (1990), has rejected the notion of women as a single category. The social model presents disabled people as an homogeneous group. Whilst this ensures that the disability studies agenda and common ground remains undisputed, such claims for a singularity can create frustration. Is there, or can there be, a unitary disability theory?

Oliver, despite the presentation of a universal model for understanding disability, draws attention to the cultural variability of disability in his 1990 monograph. There is much disagreement about the definition of disability, and the numbers of disabled people, within a particular society. As noted by Abberley (1992) in his critique of the 1988 OPCS Disability Surveys, there are key problems in developing universal definitions and concepts across societies. This is a major criticism of the WHO's first attempts at developing a classification system (Oliver 1990). The very words 'disability' and 'impairment' cannot easily be translated between European languages, let alone between Western societies and other traditions. For example, the Masai word to translate 'disabled' actually refers to a lizard that walks in an awkward way (Talle 1995). Some anthropologists have therefore pursued research which is not based on the Euro-American biomedical conceptions of disability: 'Instead of seeing impairment in terms of ability to perform specific tasks, they ask about personhood in relation to cosmology' (Ingstad and Whyte 1995, p. 37).

Disability and identity

Debates over the nature of identity and the process of identity formation have been central to the development of sociological thinking over the past twenty years. Within Marxist thought, individual identity was seen as a product of a person's class position. Whilst enlightened workers might have a clear understanding of their social position, the ruling class had a vested interest in blurring economic relations. Capitalist societies thus promulgated a range of ideologies, whose purpose was to blind working class people to the nature of their economic oppression. Oliver, in his book *The Politics of Disablement* (1990) extended this thinking to the position of disabled people, noting the way in which hegemonic culture promoted images of disabled people as either more or less than human. As well as influencing thinking within the wider society, these negative ideologies affected the thinking of disabled people themselves, limiting their sense of social and political possibilities. The disability movement, emerging during the 1970s and 80s, took on the task of raising political consciousness so that these limiting ideologies could be challenged and disabled people could develop a far more positive identity.

During the 1990s, more complex and contested theories of identity have emerged. Post-structuralist thinkers have emphasised that, far from possessing one simple fixed identity, individuals are constantly engaged in negotiating identity. Drawing on a stream of French thinking (Durkheim to Derrida), Hall (1996) appealed to a concept of identity as 'strategic and positional'. Hall's concept of identity is based on the idea of a 'violent hierarchy', so that individuals define their own identity in part by focusing on the other, on what they are not. However, because identity is always subject to negotiation rather than being fixed, it is possible for individuals and groups to revalidate a previously spurned identity, for example, homosexuals have reclaimed the term 'queer' and have reinvested it with positive rather than negative associations.

Theoretical developments in thinking about the nature of identity have had a number of practical and political implications. Identity politics have become increasingly important in the liberation struggles of oppressed groups (see Ferguson, this volume, for discussion of the ideas of Young (1990) and her critics (Fraser 1995, Phillips 1997)). Writers such as Beck (1998) argue that in post-modern society individuals have immense freedom to choose their own identity and destiny, rather than having this foisted upon them by accident of birth. On the other hand, the individualism which underpins post-structuralist and post-modernist thinking may have negative implications for the construction of a shared political vision. Unless disabled people can agree about what it means to be disabled and what the political goals of the movement should be, it may be very difficult to achieve significant progress. Struggles over cultural politics, then, far from being irrelevant, are at the heart of current debates in disability studies. Having considered some of the key issues surrounding disability, culture and identity, we now provide an overview of the structure and content of the book.

Structure and content of the book

Chapters 2, 3 and 4 (Tisdall, Watson and Priestley) address matters concerning generation, culture and identity. Tisdall focuses on the culture and identity of young disabled people. She notes that cultures of childhood/youth and disability have developed as counter-cultures, since these categories have been marginalised by the social mainstream. Young disabled people have faced multiple exclusions, lacking economic power in the same way as other children and young people, but with the additional disadvantage posed by the likelihood that in the future economic prospects might also be grim. Reviewing the traditional views of young disabled people as 'troubled', 'unformed', 'dependent', 'needy' and 'other', Tisdall argues that these negative identities have coalesced to create an overwhelmingly negative cultural perception of young disabled people. This has had real material consequences, excluding them from many aspects of citizenship and reflected in the fact that many rough sleepers and young members of the prison population have mental health problems and/or learning difficulties. Until they leave school, the lives of young disabled people are largely controlled by professionals who have great difficulty in hearing their voices. Tisdall argues for the creation of a new culture of participation, which would value the lives of young disabled people and facilitate the creation of positive rather than negative identities. Finally, the cultural diversity of young disabled people needs to be more widely acknowledged.

Nick Watson in Chapter 3 considers the ways in which disabled adults make sense of their impairments and construct their identities in everyday life. In doing so, he critiques the idea of social structures as all-powerful forces pre-determining both economic and ideological outcomes. Drawing on the stories of disabled adults, Watson argues that it is through interaction with others that identity is constantly formed, reformed and challenged. The idea of attitudinal prejudice, which tended to be played down by writers such as Oliver because of its emphasis on individuals rather than economic structures, is accorded higher priority by Watson. Whilst not denying the importance of material structures, Watson's account offers hope that social change may happen incrementally by reforming everyday cultural values.

The relationship between the cultures of age and disability is the subject of Priestley's chapter. Older people make up the majority of those identified as disabled because of the increase in impairment with age. Priestley notes that there are important commonalities in the cultural construction of old age and disability. Over the past two decades there has also been a growing awareness of the way in which

the dominant culture promotes negative images of both groups, presenting both age and disability as intrinsically deficient categories whilst
failing to acknowledge the salience of social exclusion in marginalising
both groups of people. The political struggle of older people and disabled people has involved asking questions about how things would
look if society were structured to meet their needs as a matter of priority. Despite the commonalities in cultural representations and political
struggles, most older people do not see themselves as disabled and fail
to promote the social model of disability in their thinking. Similarly,
the disabled people's movement has not sought actively to develop
links with the older people's movement, and, perhaps as a result of the
negative cultural image of old age, may have failed to acknowledge
the striking overlap of the two groups. Ultimately, Priestley argues, it is
very important for the links between the disabled people's movement
and the movement of older people to be strengthened so that a common
political agenda may be pursued.

The focus of the second section of the book is on impairment, culture
and identity, with chapters exploring the cultures of specific groups of
disabled people. Ferguson discusses the way in which people with
mental health problems construct their identities, assessing the usefulness
of notions of identity and difference in understanding the experience of
the mental health service users' movement. The terms used to describe
people with mental health problems are not innocent, but denote a range
of cultural and ideological issues which are currently being debated.
Based on individual and group discussions with eighty mental health
service users and twenty workers in fourteen mental health projects
across Central Scotland, Ferguson developed a typology of the terms
preferred by service users. The terms 'customer' and 'client', reflecting a
consumerist identity, were the least popular. 'User' and 'survivor' were
the most popular terms, suggesting activity and agency. These have
been promoted by the mental health service users' movement, in the
belief that adopting a shared identity will enable people with mental
health problems to challenge the stigmatisation and exclusion they
experience. Overall, there was considerable dissatisfaction among service users about the way in which their experiences were appropriated
and classified by others, particularly by psychiatric professionals, but
at the same time there was little agreement about preferred terminology and there did not appear to be a strong sense of a shared culture.
Ferguson considers the implications of these findings for the current
emphasis on the politics of identity, suggesting that oppressed people
should focus on the struggle for cultural recognition. Drawing on the
work of Fraser (1995, 2000), Ferguson suggests that such efforts may
militate against the development of solidarity with other groups

experiencing poverty and social exclusion. Given the difficulty of establishing a single group identity among mental health service users, efforts to emphasise the cultural difference and separateness of mental health service users from other disadvantaged people may be misplaced. Rather, energy might be better invested in making common cause with other socially exploited groups, particularly given the strong association between mental health problems and poverty.

Chapter 6 by Mairian Scott-Hill explores the relationship between deaf people and the disability movement. Whilst the disability movement has always acknowledged the distinctive concerns of deaf people, the priority has been to build a unified movement of disabled people rather than one made up of different impairment groups focusing on their specific interests. According to Scott-Hill, these attempts to develop a common identity and culture have not been particularly successful, and relations between the disability movement and the deaf people's movement continue to be fractured. Difference continues to be of major importance to deaf people, and those who use sign language see themselves as a linguistic minority oppressed by phono-centric society rather than as disabled people with impairments. Given the divisions among deaf people between those who use sign language and those who do not, and the wider rift with the disability movement over whether deafness constitutes an impairment, Scott-Hill suggests that 'a form of cultural systemic integration' represents the most fruitful path for future development.

Danny Goodley in Chapter 7 focuses on people with learning difficulties and their relationship with the wider disability movement. Like mental health service users and deaf people, those labelled as having learning difficulties do not necessarily share a common identity. In addition, their links with the wider disability movement may be tenuous, and it is certainly the case that there has sometimes been a reluctance to include fully people with learning difficulties in wider political discussion and action. Goodley explores the use of self-advocacy in assisting people with learning difficulties to develop a positive identity. Self-advocacy is seen as an alternative cultural form, able to embrace and inform a politics and culture of resistance. However, even though Goodley's interviewees see self-advocacy as an overwhelmingly positive force in their lives, some people in the disability movement regard it with some suspicion, perhaps because it involves non-disabled people as supporters and may lead to challenges to the disability movement itself, as well as the wider society.

Chapters in the third section of the book by Darke and Sweeney consider aspects of mass media and art in relation to disability and culture. Darke discusses the development of the disability arts movement. In its early stages, its aims were to challenge oppressive disablist imagery and enable disabled people to forge a new and positive culture for themselves. However, these ambitions have not been achieved. Because of its challenge to the 'great tradition' of British art, the establishment has contained it and neutralised its radicalism, concentrating funding on disability equality training and therapeutic activities. A few disabled artists have been assimilated into mainstream culture, but have often denied the political context of their work and have failed to assist other disabled people in the generation of a culture of disability. Given the power of funding state and private sponsorship to control the development of the disability arts movement, Darke is relatively pessimistic about future prospects.

The chapter by Sweeney and Riddell adopts a somewhat different perspective on disability and culture, focusing on the treatment of disability on Radio 4. Following the decision of the Controller of Radio 4 to axe *Does He Take Sugar?(DHTS?)*, the specialist programme dealing with disability issues, Sweeney undertook in-depth interviews with members of the production team in order to understand the thinking behind the decision to 'mainstream' disability. The treatment of disability on *DHTS?* was compared with the content of *You and Yours (Y & Y)*, the magazine programme which took over much of the material which had been covered in *DHTS?*. Sweeney and Riddell concluded that the project of mainstreaming is highly contentious, since there is no guarantee that disability issues will achieve serious and substantial coverage in a consumerist format. The political content of *DHTS?*, which contributed to the emergence of a culture of disability, has not been replicated on *Y & Y*. On the other hand, *Y & Y* reaches a larger audience so it is possible that a wider group of people are being made aware of disability issues. Whether the radical edge of *DHTS?* has been lost, or whether it will be maintained in other programmes run by the original production team, remains to be seen.

Chapters in the final section of the book deal with issues of cultural diversity and disability. Atkin and Hussain consider the cultural experiences of young disabled people from South Asian backgrounds, who participated in in-depth interviews with the authors. Young people from second generation South Asian families are likely to experience a range of conflicts with their parents, as they disentangle those aspects of their culture that they want to retain from those which they reject. Seeking to develop a coherent and positive identity as a disabled person is likely to further complicate the process of life transitions. Evidence from the young people suggests that the identity of being a disabled person could be used, on occasion, to challenge aspects of family culture. The young people appeared to negotiate a wide range of identities which existed alongside each other rather than within a hierarchy. As well as causing some confusion, the recognition of multiple identities was often experienced positively by the young people, who were aware of having far greater freedom than their parents had enjoyed.

Finally, the chapter by Jakubowicz and Meekosha asks the question: can multiculturalism encompass disability? The authors note that Australia is a multicultural society, although in the past this has tended to be denied. Multiculturalism has had to develop a politics of redistribution, recognising the economic oppression experienced by minority groups, and also a politics of identity, seeking to valorise the culture of groups which were previously stigmatised. Disability culture and multiculturalism have tended to exist in isolated compartments, and yet disability activists could learn a great deal from the political strategies adopted by those seeking to develop a society reflecting multicultural principles. However, the two areas cannot simply be elided because the issues facing disabled people, as well as particular impairment groups, are complex and may relate to the transient nature of some impairments. There are currently a number of political initiatives which are seeking to develop a unified approach to the economic and cultural struggles of those on the margins, underpinned by a human rights agenda. The challenge is to maintain an understanding of specific identities and cultures, whilst recognising the areas where common cause can be made.

Conclusion

In this chapter, we have outlined the themes which run throughout the book. All contributors are agreed that the oppression of disabled people has rested, in large part, on the imposition of negative and stigmatising cultural identities. The struggle for social justice, then, involves a quest for cultural recognition as well as economic redistribution. There are ongoing debates, however, about the balance to be struck between the material and the cultural arenas of political activity, with different writers in this book suggesting that one area or the other be prioritised. Within the cultural realm, we are made aware of some of the difficulties which have ensued in developing a shared disability culture. Even though the disability movement has sought to highlight the commonalities of economic oppression which transcend specific impairments, there is a constant reminder from deaf people, people with learning difficulties and mental health service users that the problems encountered and solutions sought by different groups are not the same. Whereas Deaf people already have a shared culture based on sign language, such a positive identity is far more difficult to forge for people who are mental health service users. The need for links with other groups, including older people, children and young people, and those from minority ethnic backgrounds is also a recurring theme. Often, it seems that such groups have existed in isolated compartments, failing to recognise that people do not have a single identity and oppression rarely comes from one source. An older person, for instance, may have an impairment and experience social marginalisation on account of both age and disability. There is no point in developing positive images of disabled people if older people continue to be socially devalued.

Within the book, there is a measure of both optimism and pessimism. Paul Darke, for example, suggests that the Disability Arts movement has foundered as a result of funding policies and efforts to assimilate those who might otherwise challenge the established art culture too vigorously. Sweeney and Riddell describe the demise of a progressive radio programme which played an important role in the early development of the disability movement. However, opportunities for new political alliances and campaigns in the realm of culture and identity are clearly set in many chapters of this book. It is evident that debates around disability, culture and identity, far from being played out, will continue to reverberate in coming years.

References

Abberley, P. (1992) 'Counting us out: A discussion of the OPCS Disability Surveys', *Disability, Handicap and Society*, 7, 2, pp. 139–155.

Abercrombie, N., Hill, S. and Turner, B. (1980) *Dominant ideology thesis*, Allen & Unwin, London.

Barnes, C. (1996) 'Theories of disability and the origins of oppression of disabled people in western society' in L. Barton (ed.) *Disability and Society: Emerging issues and insights*, Longman, London.

Barnes, C. and Mercer, G. (2001) 'Disability culture: Assimilation or inclusion?' in Albrecht, G., Seelman, K. and Bury, M. (eds) *Handbook of Disability Studies*, Sage, London.

Barnes, C., Mercer, G. and Shakespeare, T. (2000) *Exploring Disability: A Sociological Introduction*, Polity Press, Cambridge.

Beck, U. (1998) *Democracy without Enemies*, Polity Press, London.

Bourdieu, P. (1986) *Distinction: a social critique of the judgement of taste*, Routledge, London.

Butler, J. (1990) 'Gender Trouble, Feminist Theory and Psychoanalytic Discourse' in Nicholson, L. (ed.) *Feminism/Postmodernism*, Routledge, London.

Cambell, J. and Oliver, M. (1996) *Disability Politics: Understanding our past, changing our future*, Routledge, London.

Crawford, R. (1994) 'The boundaries of the self and the unhealthy other: Reflections on health, culture and AIDS', *Social Science and Medicine*, 38, pp. 1347–1365.

Crow, L. (1996) 'Including all of our lives' in Barnes, C. and Mercer, G. (eds) *Exploring the Divide: Illness*, Disability Press, Leeds.

Darke, P. (1998) 'Understanding cinematic representations of disability' in Shakespeare, T. (ed.) *The Disability Reader*, Cassell, London.

Davis, L. (1995) *Enforcing Normalcy: Disability, Deafness and the Body*, Verso, London.

Du Gay, P., Hall, S., James, L., Mackay, H. and Negus, K. (1997) *Doing Cultural Studies: The story of the Sony Walkman*, Sage, in association with the Open University, London.

Fraser, N. (1995) 'From Redistribution to Recognition? Dilemmas of Justice in a "Post-Socialist" Age, *New Left Review*, **212**, pp. 68–92.

Fraser, N. (2000) 'Rethinking recognition' in *New Left Review*, **3**, pp. 107–220.

Fraser, N. and Nicholson, L. (1990) 'Social criticism without philosophy: an encounter between feminism and postmodernism' in L. Nicholson (ed.) *Feminism/Postmodernism*, Routledge, London.

Friedman, J. (1994) *Cultural Identity and Global Processes*, Sage, London.

Fuss, D. (1989) *Essentially speaking: feminism, nature and difference*, Routledge, London.

Hall, S. (1996) 'Introduction: Who needs identity' in Hall, S. and du Gay, P. (eds) *Questions of Cultural Identity?*, Sage, London.

Hevey, D. (1992) *The Creatures Time Forgot: Photography and Disability Imagery*, Routledge, London.

Ingstad, B. and Whyte, S. (eds) (1995) *Disability and Culture*, University of California Press, Berkeley.

Karpf, A. (1988) *Doctoring the Media*, Routledge, Kegan Paul, London.

Keith, L. (2000) *Take up thy bed and walk*, Women's Press, London.

Norden, M. (1994) *The Cinema of Isolation: A history of disability in the movies*, Rutgers University Press, New Brunswick, NJ.

Oliver, M. (1990) *The Politics of Disablement*, Macmillan, Basingstoke.

Oliver, M. (1996) *Understanding Disability: From Theory to Practice*, Macmillan, Basingstoke.

Phillips, A. (1997) 'From inequality to difference: a severe case of displacement', *New Left Review*, **224**, pp. 143–153.

Pinder, R. (1995) 'Bringing back the body without the blame?: the experience of ill and disabled people at work', *Sociology of Health and Illness*, 17: 605–31.

Pinder, R. (1996) 'Sick-but-fit or fit-but-sick? Ambiguity and identity at the workplace' in Barnes, C. and Mercer, G. (eds) *Exploring the Divide: Illness and disability*, Disability Press, Leeds.

Scheper-Hughes, N. and Lock, M. (1987) 'The mindful body: A prolegomenon to work in medical anthropology', *Medical Anthropology Quarterly*, **1**, pp. 6–41.

Schutz, A. (1970) *On Phenomenology and Social Relations*, University of Chicago Press, Chicago.

Shakespeare, T. (1994) 'Cultural Representation of Disabled People: Dustbins for disavowal', *Disability, Handicap and Society*, **9** (3), pp. 283–301.

Shakespeare, T. (1996) 'Disability, Identity and Difference' in Barnes, C. and Mercer, C. (eds) *Exploring the Divide: Illness and Disability*, Disability Press, Leeds.

Shakespeare, T., Gillespie-Sells, K. and Davies, D. (1996) *The Sexual Politics of Disability*, Cassell, London.

Swain, J., Finkelstein, V., French, S. and Oliver, M. (1994) *Disabling Barriers – Enabling Environments*, Sage, London.

Talle, A. (1995) 'A Child is a Child: Disability and Equality Among the Kenya Masai' in Williams, R. (1976/1988) *Keywords: A vocabulary of culture and society*, Fontana, London.

Thomas, C. (1999) Female Forms: Experiencing and Understanding Disability, Open University Press, Milton Keynes.

Turner, B. and Roject, C. (2001) *Society and Culture (Theory, Culture & Society)*, Sage, London.

Williams, R. (1981) *Culture*, Fontana, London.

Williams, R. (1989) *Resources of Hope*, Verso, London.

Williams, Y. (1976/1988) *Keywords: a vocabulary of culture and society*, Fontana, London.

Young, I. M. (1990) *Justice and the Politics of Difference*, Princeton University Press, Princeton NJ.

CHAPTER 2

A culture of participation?

E. Kay M. Tisdall

I find that the Government doesn't consult us as disabled people. They make our decisions for us . . . I think it's about time they started consulting us, we have a voice, we need to come out with our voices.

I think they [the Government] are just starting to take us seriously . . . some of them are starting to realise that some of the decisions they make do affect us, so they want to do what is best for us.

(Two young people quoted in Article 12 (1999), p. 36)

The UK has been much criticised for not having a culture of listening to children, young people or disabled people, and of failing to involve them in key decisions that affect them (e.g. Coles 1995; Lansdown 1995; Oliver 1996). Young disabled people – who may at times be considered 'dependent children', at others 'troubled adolescents' or 'needy disabled people' – may be particularly at risk of being excluded from participation and community membership.

The exclusion of young disabled people has been a long-standing policy-research concern in the UK, framed predominantly as the 'transitional problem' from school to work or school to 'adulthood'. From Ferguson and Kerr (1955 and 1958) to recent studies (Mitchell 1999; Riddell *et al.* 1999), research has traced the difficulties many young disabled people face. For example, in 1994 Hirst and Baldwin produced *Unequal Opportunities: Growing Up Disabled,* based on interviews with 591 disabled young people (aged 14–22) and a comparison group of 726 young people. The findings are sadly familiar: 'a sizeable minority of disabled young people, we estimate between 30 and 40 per cent, would find great difficulty in attaining a degree of independence in adult life comparable to that of young people in the general population'

(p. 110). Young people who were 'severely and multiply disabled' were particularly disadvantaged. These conclusions are based on examining a host of different aspects of young people's lives: employment, education, income, self-esteem and sense of personal control, living arrangements, social lives including friendships and leisure activities, and contacts with health and social services.

Hirst and Baldwin's (1994) research in many ways typifies the more recent research for young disabled people, albeit with a more extensive survey than most. They have moved away from the past preoccupation with employment as the key indicator of adult status, to include other aspects. They compare young disabled people with their non-disabled peers, concluding that young disabled people are substantially more disadvantaged (the 'transitional problem'). The implicit goal is 'independence', which is correlated with, if not required as, a definition of 'adulthood' but beginning to be questioned. The importance of young disabled people themselves being involved in decisions that affect them has gained prominence and was noted in the book's recommendations.

Just as arguments for participation became increasingly prominent in the 1990s' transitional literature on young disabled people, the late 1990s saw the introduction of the concept of 'inclusion'. For example, the Beattie Committee's report on Post-School Education and Training of Young People with Special Needs takes 'inclusiveness' as its organising principle: '. . . Inclusiveness means that the needs, abilities and aspirations of young people should be recognised, understood and met within a supportive environment which encourages them to achieve their goals and to make real, measurable progress' (Beattie Report 1999, p. 10). According to the report, this principle was deliberately chosen to avoid a 'deficit' model implied by definitions of 'needs' or 'problems'.

The concept of 'social inclusion' more broadly has become part of UK and European policy rhetoric. Perhaps because it has become a popularised policy concept, its exact definition is elusive. Tony Blair, the UK Prime Minister, has described social exclusion as:

> a short-hand label for what can happen when individuals or areas suffer from a combination of linked problems such as unemployment, poor skills, low incomes, poor housing, high crime environments, bad health and family breakdown.
> (quoted on Scottish Social Inclusion Network (SIN) web-site)

Those writing on social exclusion have made a distinction between the concept and poverty or multiple deprivation, with the former including more 'qualitative, intangible and abstract elements such as depression, low self-esteem and isolation' (Stevens *et al.* 1999, p. 3). It can be seen as a dynamic rather than static concept, emphasising processes in society that disadvantage individuals, groups and communities. Social exclusion/inclusion at least has the potential to emphasise society's barriers rather than individual failings. And, argue Stevens and colleagues, social inclusion is fundamentally about participation: 'Participation can be thought of as the opposite to the process of social exclusion' (1999, p. 3). With such ideas, social inclusion links up neatly with recent theorisations of citizenship (e.g. Lister 1998).

T.H. Marshall's seminal lecture on 'citizenship' defines citizenship as:

> ... a status bestowed on those who are full members of a community. All who possess the status are equal with respect to the rights and duties with which the status is endowed.   (Marshall 1963, p. 87)

Marshall describes the historical evolution of 'citizenship' in the gradual accumulation of civil, political and finally social rights. No doubt due to its impact, the lecture has attracted considerable critique and thus led to development of the concept of 'citizenship'. Of particular interest for this chapter, Marshall's theorisation is accused of underestimating the *process* and *practice* of citizenship in his emphasis on the *status* of citizenship (see, for example, Lister 1997).

Are young disabled people included in the status, process and practices of *citizenship*, and thus *included* in their communities? This chapter will explore this question, by considering the three different academic and research literatures on childhood, youth and disability. It will argue that, by being defined as 'other' to an adult or a non-disabled person, all three identities lead to possible exclusion from citizenship and rights. It will conclude by asking whether the rhetoric of participation and recent emphases on rights and citizenship have the potential to create a 'culture of inclusion' and thus change the way policy-makers/researchers/the literature/adults both conceptualise the 'transitional problem' and perceive young disabled people.

'Dependent children'

Until very recently, much of the 'childhood' literature was actually a literature on how adults viewed children (Shamgar-Handelman 1994).

Traditional theories, such as Parsons' socialisation theory and Piagetian child development, see adults as mature, rational and competent whereas children are viewed as 'less than fully human, unfinished or incomplete' (Jenks 1996, p. 10). Childhood, the 'new sociologists of childhood' argue, has been wrongly seen as natural, 'an enduring, historically consistent and universal' construct (Goldson 1997, p. 19), which has been defined as the *absence* of adulthood. The very social construct of childhood, therefore, is dependent on the construct of adulthood.

Qvortrup makes the explicit connection between this social construct of childhood as 'human becomings' rather than 'human beings' and the exclusion of children:

> ...adulthood is regarded as the goal and end-point of individual development or perhaps even the very meaning of a person's childhood. They are however revealing for the maybe unintended message, which seems to indicate that children are not members or at least not integrated members of society. This attitude, while perceiving childhood as a moratorium and a preparatory phase, thus confirms postulates about children as 'naturally' incompetent and incapable.
>
> (Qvortrup 1994, p. 2)

From such constructions come arguments that children are not citizens and, further, they do not even have rights because they lack rationality, they lack competence, they need protection not autonomy, and they must be socialised into 'good citizens' (see, for example, Phillips 1997; Purdy 1992). Children are seen as irrational because they either lack the competence to be rational or lack the experience or understanding to be so. Much of the recent childhood research has sought to counter such arguments, demonstrating the fuller extent of children's competency and rationality than previously found (e.g. Alderson 2000, Mayall 2001).

Not only are the *constructs* of childhood and adulthood dependent on each other but the *content* of their relationship is the dependency of children on adults (Shamgar-Handelman 1994). For example, until recently in UK law, children were perceived as the property of their parents. A great deal of legislation still relies on parents to protect and promote the 'rights', or best interests, of the children. Children rarely receive benefits directly, under the age of 16, but their mothers (i.e. child benefit) or parents (i.e. income support, most tax credits) do. Moss and

Petrie (1997) describe a dominant discourse about children in the UK, that sees children as the private responsibility of their parents, as passive dependents of parents and recipients of services, and parents as the consumers of marketised services for children.

The consequences of these common constructs of childhood can be traced in the citizenship literature. Lister argues against 'equating dependency with weakness and incapacity for citizenship' (1997, p. 108). Yet her description of young people's transition to the rights and responsibilities of adult citizenship (p. 76) does not seem to allow for children and young people to be citizens now, but only in the future. This is stated more explicitly in earlier writing:

> Although they are members of the community, children are not full citizens in the sense of political and legal rights which pertain to citizenship; the social rights of citizenship come to them indirectly through the adults responsible for their care.   (Lister 1990, p. 62)

It is worth noting that Lister does not extensively consider child or youth citizenship and, by her 1997 book, does cite the United Nations Convention on the Rights of the Child. But she does not attribute citizenship to children. Thus, while potentially having rights, children are excluded from 'full membership' of their communities and instead cast as dependents on their carers.

'Troubled adolescents'

While recognising the social construction of children as 'human becomings' is relatively new, 'youth' has quintessentially been theorised as a time of transition. At least three strands can be traced, in psychology, cultural studies and transitional research. The dominant psychological account has focused on the 'troubled adolescent'. For example, Coleman and Hendry (1990) describe an upsurge of instincts at puberty and the inadequacies of psychological defences. Further, stresses and tensions caused by external pressures on the adolescent can seriously threaten the smooth path to an adult identity. Erikson (1963) argues that children need to emerge from childhood with a definite sense of who they are. He characterises youth as often a period of role confusion which usually leads on to clear ideas about function (occupational identity), beliefs (ideological identity) and sex role (sexual identity). Another strand of youth studies has been the influence of the Centre for Contemporary Cultural Studies (University of Birmingham), which investigates youth cultures. Willis' (1977) ethnographic study of working class 'lads' in school remains a key text for youth research today, demonstrating the lads' active involvement in schooling's social reproduction of their adult working lives. Other work has concentrated on youth (sub)cultures in terms of 'style' and peer groups, with recent attention to the youth identities being defined largely by consumerism and consuming (e.g. Miles 1998; Widdicombe and Woofit 1995). The third strand has paralleled the transitional literature on young disabled people (although seemingly with next to complete disregard for it: see Tisdall 2001a), in its concern about the 'transitional problem' for young people in reaching adult status. Research in the 1980s focused on 'transitions' and then 'trajectories': 'the use of the term trajectory implying that labour market destinations were largely determined by social forces and transitions largely outside the control of individual social actors' (Evans and Furlong 1997, pp. 1–2). The structural approach became unpopular with some in the 1990s, with the influence of 'post-structuralist' and 'post-modernist' thinking. Theorisation around young people's individual agency, and the ways individuals assessed risk and negotiated opportunities, predominated (e.g. Beck 1992) but there were also those who sought to combine both structuralism and individualised risk (e.g. Coles 1995; Furlong and Cartmel 1997).

What is common to all three strands of youth studies is their focus on young people as *becoming* adults, seeing youth *in contrast* to adulthood (as well as childhood). The psychological and trajectory/transition/risk strands all perceive youth as in transition, as precariously balanced between childhood and adulthood. The youth culture studies provide a more proactive version of youth but, with a strong focus on youth subcultures, also 'other' than adult. None of these approaches lead to perceiving youth *as* citizens (for more discussion, see France 1996; Tisdall 2001a).

'Needy disabled people'

The concept of disability 'culture' is more new to theorisation and its various possibilities and dimensions discussed throughout this book. The tradition of disability studies has been a focus on the 'social model of disability' in contrast to the past medicalisation of disability. The seminal UK works in disability studies theorise 'disability' as a creation of the capitalist mode of production, with disabled people defined as non-productive in the work force and dominant ideologies (e.g. Oliver 1990). While disabled people may have an impairment, their disability is created by the barriers society creates and imposes. Disability studies academics such as Shakespeare (1994) have looked at the prejudicial views engendered by how disabled people have been represented as 'other' throughout history. Just as childhood and youth is defined by its contrast to adulthood, disability is defined against a 'norm' of being able-bodied.

Oliver explicitly traces how disabled people have been systematically excluded from citizenship. Linking to Marshall's three categories of rights, he describes how disabled people are denied such civil rights as the right to use public space (due to inaccessibility), political rights such as the ability to access polling booths or accessible information, and social rights such as an adequate standard of living. He provides particular insights into the irony of what are (at least superficially) intended to be 'social rights' provided by a state welfare system actually subordinating disabled people:

> ... professionalised service provision within a needs-based system of welfare has added to existing forms of discrimination and in addition, has created new forms of its own including the provision of stigmatised services such as day care and the development of professional assessments ...
>
> (1996, pp. 75–6)

In such ways, state welfare has not only failed to ensure the citizenship rights of disabled people but in fact has infringed or taken away some of these rights (p. 52).

Defined as 'the other'?

Citizenship is a concept arguably based on the inclusion of some and the exclusion of others (Oliver 1996; Tisdall 1994) – it depends how widely the boundaries are drawn. The 'othering' of particular groups, due to identities which supersede any others they may have, frequently places these groups on the outside of that boundary. A great deal of writing on citizenship has argued against such 'othering', for women (Lister 1997), for disabled people (Oliver 1996), for children (Knutsson 1996) or for youth (France 1996), to assert that these groups should be considered citizens.

Certain of the commonalities across these literatures are striking and certain literatures could learn from an angle particularly developed in others. For example, the discussion above has traced the 'othering' based on dependence. This 'othering' through dependence directly relates to exclusion from citizenship. Citizens not only have equal rights, but equal duties, to follow Marshall's quotation earlier in this chapter. If people are only recipients of other people's duty-obligations, they become outwith the boundaries of citizenship. Disability studies (in common with feminist studies) has been particularly critical of the dichotomy between dependence and independence, based on the presumption of 'productive' waged employment. Writers such as Morris (1993) have argued for some time for the recognition of people's interdependence. Research on caring demonstrates how caring and (in)dependence belong on a continuum, with disabled people often taking on roles of caring and being cared for (Morris 1993; Walmsley 1993). The focus on 'physical' (in)dependence has been challenged, with advocates for independent living arguing that independence is about making choices and decisions and not whether the person can enact them him/herself (e.g. Morris 1993). Very recent childhood studies have also criticised the idea that children are non-contributors to their families and society. Research has traced the extent to which children do contribute to their families, emotionally, practically and sometimes economically (e.g. Brannen et al. 2000, Mayall 2001). International research has reminded northern countries that their childhood construct is not universal and that children in southern countries are often expected to take a much more active role in their household economy (e.g. Punch 2000). Debates about 'young carers' have brought together childhood and disability studies to break down notions of dependence (e.g. Olsen 2000). Youth studies, to a large extent, remains the 'outlier'. Prominent conceptualisations of youth transitions continue to posit transitions between dependence and independence (for discussion and examples, see Tisdall 2001a).

Both the childhood and disability literatures have explored the 'institutionalisation' of their respective groups, and the ways by which these have excluded children and disabled people from participation in their communities. Children are increasingly institutionalised, according to Qvortrup (1994), not only in schools but also through day care (Smith and Barker 2000) and formalised leisure activities (McKendrick et al. 2000). Indeed, Mayall (2001) argues that it is in such public spaces where children are most excluded:

In two of the major settings of their daily lives, public spaces and school, they are assigned moral incompetence. Thus UK children, and perhaps especially city children, are largely excluded from decision-making outside the home. Indeed, the two main arenas where they are able to enact competence are in the family and in peer relationships . . . and these arenas are obscured from public view and therefore from public understanding. (p. 125)

With the medicalisation of disability, many disabled people were sent to residential and/or segregated institutions both as adults and children. While mainstreaming in schools and community care may have disaggregated some of this segregation, young people may be 'mainstreamed' in segregated units attached to mainstream schools:

I went to a mainstream school but I was still segregated because I was put into a special class . . . I wasn't allowed to take part because I was special, I was segregated. [For example] someone in my year was dealing with drugs and everyone in my year was interviewed apart from me because I was in a special class. I was treated as innocent because they believed I wouldn't have anything to do with it.
(young person quoted in Article 12 (1999), p. 33)

The continual cycle of training for (young and then not so young) adult disabled people may be just another form of warehousing (Baron *et al.* 1999). The criticism of youth institutionalisation is less common to youth studies but elements of it can be drawn out. Large proportions of young people are imprisoned. Crime does peak in youth but self-report surveys show that a lower proportion of adults who report offending are caught by the police let alone imprisoned (Graham and Bowling 1995). Furstenberg (2000) notes the irony of the various social institutions that isolate young people (i.e. further/higher education, youth training) while proposing to prepare the young people for their future adult roles in the community. Part of the institutionalisation experience is invariably professional surveillance.

If children, disabled people or young people are not in institutions, in various ways they are explicitly or implicitly excluded from public space – a very direct exclusion from 'public' citizenship. Disabled people with a variety of impairments are still very practically excluded due to inaccessibility (even though the Disability Discrimination Act 1995 has sought to address such discrimination). Children are 'familialised'

(Qvortrup 1994), ideologically and often practically, and thus expected to be with their families, in their home. Research on childhood has much criticised the reduced mobility of children in the UK, created by a combination of parental fears and increased adult dominance of so-called public space (e.g. Valentine 1996). Research with children and young people has demonstrated the value many place, both male and female, on space 'on the streets'. While for adults this might be considered 'public space', for some young people without private bedrooms and spacious homes, it may be the only 'private' space where they can be with their friends (Matthews *et al.* 2000). Yet, the idea that younger children on the street are in danger and older children/young people are threats and disruptive has led to both informal and formal curfews, with police patrolling and taking children/young people back to their homes.

If such exclusion from citizenship can be traced for many children, disabled people and young people, these can be demonstrated as coming together for young disabled people. Research has demonstrated that a disproportionate number of imprisoned young people have mental health problems and/or learning difficulties (Audit Commission 1996). If these young people are out on the street, they may be the ones stopped by the police and considered the 'trouble makers'. Young disabled people – until they fall out of the service structure when they leave school – are typically controlled by professional judgements and expectations, with a range of professionals involved in their lives (for discussion, see Davis and Watson 2001). The typical cycle of job training and further education sometimes combined with day centres, particularly for young people with learning difficulties (Baron *et al.* 1999), maintains their institutionalisation and segregation. Hirst and Baldwin (1994) and Cavet (1998) demonstrate the exclusion of many disabled young people from leisure and recreation activities, frequently having to rely on their parents for social activities and being less likely to attend typical youth venues such as cinemas and discos. Positively, young disabled people are now criticising their exclusion; negatively, such experiences are invariably revealed when young disabled people are consulted:

> People think that if you can't speak properly you can't take part.
>
> People talk to you as if you're deaf – they talk to the person beside you instead of to you directly.
>
> We get treated like babies, patted, patronised.
>
> (Young disabled people quoted in Save the Children Fund Scotland 1999, p. 47)

Is it possible to have a culture of participation?

The chapter up to now has largely focused on the negative, the ways by which three identities of young disabled people can and often do lead to their exclusion from participation, citizenship and thus their community membership. The above critical analysis, however, has been the platform for agitating for change. While it has limitations, the Disability Discrimination Act 1995 was the first UK civil rights legislation for disabled people. Disabled people have organised themselves into powerful movements, whose voices can be strongly heard in the media and political circles. International conventions and statements have been made in relation to disabled people's rights (e.g. Standard Rules on the Equalization of Opportunities for Persons with Disabilities, resolution 48/96, UN General Assembly 1993). The traditional or dominant constructions of childhood have been contrasted with alternatives, which recognise children as agents, as societal members, as holders of rights. The United Nations Convention on the Rights of the Child has been almost universally accepted across the world. Legislation is changing, so that children's rights are being incorporated into law, such as the obligation on education to take account of children's views in significant decisions recently introduced to Scottish children's law (see Tisdall 2001b for more discussion). Children and young people are being increasingly consulted on policies. Various structures are being created, such as Youth Parliaments and Children's Commissioners, to put more power behind young people's and children's views.

Certainly in the UK, there is ever-increasing political and professional rhetoric about participation in 'public' decision-making. Service planning now regularly needs to demonstrate that service users have been consulted. Training sessions abound on how to 'listen to children'. Organisations and initiatives of young people are growing in number, where young people set the agenda and control (within the limitations of the law) the finances. Arguments are being made that young disabled people must be part of this new 'culture of participation'. Their participation should not be based solely on disability questions but they should be involved, with other young people, in all the kinds of decisions that affect their lives (e.g. Children in Scotland 2002). However, the very public institution frequently used to access young disabled people's views – schools – can be the very institution least likely to have a culture of participation. Young people do report frustration with the current adult enthusiasm with their participation, criticising it as too frequently tokenistic and cursory (Garumurthy 2000). One young disabled person

spoke of his experience at school, when he wanted to challenge a decision: 'You can tell when they are [listening] and when they are not.
Quite a lot of teachers do not listen deeply.' (Children in Scotland 2002,
p. 13). A 'culture of participation' may be growing but its actualisation
may not always be delivering on its rhetoric.

Partially because of such experiences, both positive and negative,
conceptualisations of participation are becoming more sophisticated.
Foundational in its time, the limitations of Hart's 'ladder of participation' are being discovered. Hart (1992) adapted Arnstein's model of
citizen participation, which ranks projects by means of a 'ladder of participation'. There are eight levels of participation on the ladder ranging
from 'manipulative' to 'child-initiated'. Hart's ladder seems to imply
that the 'best' participation is always on the highest rung: Green (1999)
questions this implication, saying that choice is the key measure for participation in a project. Some children and young people may not wish to
take full direction but may rather wish adults to listen to their opinions
and take them into account. As Willow (1997) argues, there is no one
way of involving children and young people and methods must be
tailored to the needs and priorities of those involved.

The limits of 'participation' are also being articulated. Murray and
Hallett (2000) note that it is no coincidence that 'the right to participate
is often discussed in relation to the least powerful in society' (p. 15).
They note that the right to participation: '. . . almost invariably exists in
the absence of another right, that of the right to self-determination, and
could therefore be described as a "cosmetic" or "compensatory" right'
(p. 15). The adults can remain the powerful ones who consult while the
young people remain the powerless who are consulted (Cairns 2001).
A culture of participation can still be a culture of control.

All three areas of policy/literature have been criticised for ignoring
diversity due to such characteristics as gender, ethnicity, geography,
age/stage, type of impairment, sexual orientation etc. (e.g. Morris 1993;
James, Jenks and Prout 1998). Yet, even the critics do still draw on
the broader categories of childhood, disability and youth – or young
disabled people. Perhaps the test of the above changes in creating a
more participative, inclusive society will be when it will no longer seem
sensible to so group such heterogeneous people together, for either
theoretical analysis or political lobbying against discrimination.

● References

Alderson, P. (2000) *Young Children's Rights. Exploring beliefs, principles and practice*, Jessica Kingsley, London.

Article 12 (1999) *Respect! A report into how well Article 12 of the UN Convention on the Rights of the Child is put into practice across the UK*, Nottingham: Article 12.

Audit Commission (1996) *Misspent Youth: Young People and Crime*, Abingdon: Audit Commission Publications.

Baron, S., Riddell, S. and Wilson, S. (1999) 'The Secret of Eternal Youth: identity, risk and learning difficulties', *British Journal of Sociology of Education*, **20**(4), pp. 483–499.

Beattie Report (1999) *Implementing Inclusiveness: Realising Potential*, Scottish Executive, Edinburgh.

Beck, U. (1992) *The Risk Society: towards a new modernity*, Sage, London.

Brannen, J., Heptinstall, E. and Bhopal, K. (2000) *Connecting Children*, Routledge/Falmer Press, London.

Cairns, L. (2001) 'Investing in Children: Learning How to Promote the Rights of All Children', *Children & Society*, **15**, pp. 347–360.

Cavet, J. (1998) 'Leisure and Friendship' in Robinson, C. and Stalker, K. (eds) *Growing Up with Disability*, Jessica Kingsley Publishers, London.

Children in Scotland (2002) *What matters to me!*, Children in Scotland, Edinburgh.

Coleman, J.C. and Hendry, L. (1990) *The Nature of Adolescence*, 2nd edn, Routledge, London.

Coles, B. (1995) *Youth and Social Policy: Youth citizenship and youth careers*, UCL Press, London.

Davis, J. and Watson, N. (2001) 'Where are the children's experiences? Analysing social and cultural exclusion in "special" and "mainstream" schools', *Disability & Society*, **16**(5), pp. 671–687.

Erikson, E.H. (1963) *Childhood and Society*, Penguin, Harmondsworth.

Evans, K. and Furlong, A. (1997) 'Metaphors of youth transitions: niches, pathways, trajectories or navigations' in Bynner, J., Chisholm, L. and Furlong, A. (eds) *Youth, citizenship and social change in a European context*, Avebury, Aldershot.

Ferguson, T. and Kerr, A.W. (1955) 'After-histories of girls educated in special schools for mentally-handicapped children', *Glasgow Medical Journal*, **36**, pp. 50–56.

Ferguson, T. and Kerr, A.W. (1958) 'After-histories of boys educated in special schools for mentally-handicapped children', *Scottish Medical Journal*, **3**, pp. 31–38.

France, A. (1996) 'Youth and Citizenship in the 1990s', *Youth & Policy*, **53**, pp. 28–43.

Furlong, A. and Cartmel, F. (1997) *Young People and Social Change*, Open University Press, Buckingham.

Furstenberg, F.F. (2000) 'The Sociology of Adolescence and Youth in the 1990s: A Critical Commentary', *Journal of Marriage and the Family*, **62**, pp. 895–910.

Garumurthy, R. (2000) 'Next Steps: The Carnegie Young People Initiative 2000–02' in Frost, R. (ed.) *Voices Unheard: Young People at the Beginning of the 21st Century*, Youth Work Press, London.

Goldson, B. (1997) 'Childhood: An Introduction to Historical and Theoretical Analysis' in Scraton, P. (ed.) *Childhood in Crisis?*, UCL Press, London.

Graham, J. and Bowling, B. (1995) *Young People and Crime*, HMSO, London.

Green, D.R. (1999) 'Political Participation of Youth in the United Kingdom' in Riepl, B. and Wintersberger, H. (eds) *Political Participation of Youth below Voting Age*, European Centre, Vienna.

Hart, R.A. (1992) *Children's Participation: from tokenism to citizenship*, UNICEF International Child Development Centre, Geneva.

Hirst, M. and Baldwin, S. (1994) *Unequal Opportunities: Growing Up Disabled*, Social Policy Research Unit, HMSO, London.

James, A., Jenks, C. and Prout, A. (1998) *Theorizing Childhood*, Polity Press, Cambridge.

Jenks, C. (1996) *Childhood*, Routledge, London.

Knutsson, K.E. (1996) 'A new vision of childhood' in Jeleff, S. (ed.) *The Child as Citizen*, Council of Europe Publishing, Belgium.

Lansdown, G. (1995) *Taking Part: Children's participation in decision-making*, IPPR, London.

Lister, R. (1990) *The Exclusive Society: Citizenship and the Poor*, CPAG, London.

Lister, R. (1997) *Citizenship: Feminist Perspectives*, Macmillan, London.

Lister, R. (1998) 'Citizenship on the margins: Citizenship, social work and social action', *European Journal of Social Work*, 1(1), pp. 5–18.

Marshall, T.H. (1963) 'Citizenship and Social Class' in *Sociology at the Crossroads and Other Essays*, Heinemann, London.

Matthews, H., Limb, M. and Taylor, M. (2000) 'The "Street as Thirdspace"', in Holloway, S.L. and Valentine, G. (eds) *Children's Geographies: playing, living and learning*, Routledge, London.

Mayall, B. (2001) 'Understanding childhoods: a London study', in Alanen, L. and Mayall, B. (eds) *Conceptualizing Child-Adult Relations*, Routledge/Falmer, London.

McKendrick, J.H., Bradford, M.G. and Fielder, A.V. (2000) 'Time for a Party! Making sense of commercialisation of leisure space for children' in Holloway, S.L. and Valentine, G. (eds) *Children's Geographies: playing, living and learning*, Routledge, London.

Miles, S. (1998) *Consumerism – as a way of life*, Sage Publications, London.

Mitchell, W. (1999) 'Leaving Special School: the next step and future aspirations', *Disability & Society*, 14(6), pp. 753–769.

Morris, J. (1993) *Independent Lives: Community Care and Disabled People*, Macmillan, London.

Moss, P. and Petrie, P. (1997) *Children's services: the need for a new approach*. A discussion paper. Thomas Coram Research Unit, Institute of Education University of London, London.

Murray, C. and Hallett, C. (2000) 'Young People's Participation in Decisions affecting their Welfare', *Childhood*, 7(1), pp. 11–25.

Oliver, M. (1990) *The Politics of Disablement*, Macmillan, London.

Oliver, M. (1996) *Understanding Disability: From Theory to Practice*, Macmillan, Basingstoke.

Olsen, R. (2000) 'Families under the microscope: parallels between the young carers debate of the 1990s and the transformation of childhood in the late nineteenth century', *Children & Society*, 14, pp. 384–394.

Phillips, M. (1997) *All Must Have Prizes*, Warner Books, London.

Punch, S. (2000) 'Children's Strategies for Creating Playspaces: Negotiating independence in rural Bolivia' in Holloway, S.L. and Valentine, G. (eds) *Children's Geographies: playing, living and learning*, Routledge, London.

Purdy, L.M. (1992) *In Their Best Interest? The Case against Equal Rights for Children*, Cornell University Press, Ithaca and London.

Riddell, S., Wilson, S. and Baron, S. (1999) 'Captured customers: people with learning difficulties in the social market', *British Educational Research Journal*, 25(4), pp. 445–461.

Qvortrup, J. (1994) 'Childhood Matters: An Introduction' in Qvortrup, J., Bardy, M., Sgritta, G. and Wintersberger, H. (eds) *Childhood Matters. Social Theory, Practice and Politics*, Avebury, Aldershot.

Save the Children Fund Scotland (1999) *Our Lives*, SCF Scotland, Edinburgh.

Scottish Social Inclusion Network http://www.scotland.gov.uk/inclusion/whatis.htm accessed 9.12.98.

Shakespeare, T. (1994) 'Cultural Representation of Disabled People – Dustbins for Disavowal', *Disability & Society*, 9(3), pp. 283–299.

Shamgar-Handelman, L. (1994) 'To Whom Does Childhood Belong?' in Qvortrup, J., Bardy, M., Sgritta, G. and Wintersberger, H. (eds) *Childhood Matters. Social Theory, Practice and Politics*, Avebury, Aldershot.

Smith, F. and Barker, J. (2000) '"Out of school", in school: a social geography of out of school childcare' in Holloway, S.L. and Valentine, G. (eds) *Children's Geographies: playing, living and learning*, Routledge, London.

Stevens, A., Bur, A. and Young, L. (1999) 'Partial, Unequal and Conflictual: Problems in Using Participation for Social Inclusion in Europe', *Social Work in Europe*, 6(2), pp. 2–9.

Tisdall, E.K.M. (1994) 'Why not consider Citizenship? A critique of post-school transitional models for young disabled people', *Disability and Society*, 9(1), pp. 3–17.

Tisdall, K. (2001a) 'Failing to make the transition? Theorisation of the "transition to adulthood" for young disabled people' in Priestley, M. (ed.) *Disability and the Life Course*, Cambridge University Press, Cambridge.

Tisdall, K. (2001b) 'Social Inclusion or Exclusion? Recent policy trends in Scottish children's services for disabled children' in Riddell, S. and Tett, L. (eds) *Education, Social Justice and Inter-agency Working: Joined up or fracture policy?*, Routledge, London.

Valentine, G. (1996) 'Children should be seen and not heard: the production and transgression of adults' public space', *Urban Geography*, 17(3), pp. 205–220.

Walmsley, J. (1993) 'Contradictions in caring: reciprocity and interdependence', *Disability, Handicap and Society*, 8, pp. 129–141.

Widdicombe, S. and Woofit, R. (1995) *The Language of youth subcultures. Social identity in action*, Harvester Wheatsheaf, London.

Willis, P. (1977) *Learning to labour: how working class kids get working class jobs*, Gower, Aldershot.

Willow, C. (1997) *Hear! Hear!*, Local Government Information Unit, London.

CHAPTER 3

Daily denials: The routinisation of oppression and resistance

Nick Watson

Introduction

> Those we meet cannot fail to notice our disablement even if they turn away and avoid thinking about us afterwards. An impaired and deformed body is a 'difference' that hits everyone hard at first. Inevitably it produces an instinctive revulsion, has a disturbing effect. Our own first reaction to this is to want to hide ourselves in the crowd, to attempt to buy acceptance on any terms, to agree uncritically with whatever is the done thing. (Hunt 1998, p. 12)

This chapter documents disabled people's accounts, drawn from semi-structured interviews, of their interaction with non-disabled people and the social and physical environment in which they live. It is in these encounters that, as Goffman (1979) puts it, 'most of the world's work gets done'. Whilst, sociologically speaking, social institutions, relationships, social structures, organisations, social change, social movements and so on provide the subject matter for a sociology of disability, these emerge through the conduct of individuals. It is only through abstractions of such conduct that these structures are made manifest. Structures are, like all our knowings and all our creations, underpinned by meanings and values, the stuff of culture. Cultures can thus be seen as essential elements within social structures (Bourdieu 1998). These structures are experienced not as facts, but as outcomes. Social structures do not exist outside of the sociological imagination. So Lemert writes:

> ...social structures are by their very nature re-constructions of reality
> after the fact. No one ever encounters the reality of structures as such
> – not markets, not states, not stratification systems. Real people, rather,
> encounter insufficient pay checks, impossibly excluding bureaucratic
> rules, and particular slights and injuries, but not the structures
> themselves. The reality of social structures is always, unavoidably,
> composed in the sociological imagination...   (1997, p. 74)

Structures are perceived as the product of discourse, occurring in language and through social interaction. Social structures are contingent and invented, they do not rest on a solid foundation, but are open to change, to local reading, to reinvention. To discuss social structures without examining the language, the signs, the images through which structures emerge is to suggest that structures exist as some form of social reality, some tangible product that can be seen and felt. Elias' (1994) work on the changing nature of civilisation and the social construction of what is considered civilised, for example, clearly shows how these structures are continuously being destroyed and reinvented.

In the quotation from Paul Hunt at the start of this chapter, he makes it clear that it is through interactions with others that he becomes aware of his bodily difference and that this awareness affects his behaviour. This is also a central theme of Jenny Morris' *Pride Against Prejudice* and some of the work of Lois Keith (1996). Both Morris and Keith argue that the prejudice experienced by disabled people in their day-to-day interactions with non-disabled people lies at the very heart of segregation and oppression and that it is necessary to understand disabled people's views and accounts of their daily round of social interaction. Through this an understanding of the patterns of cultural and social oppression of disabled people, of the challenges faced by disabled people and the structures that impact on their lives can be unpacked and interpreted.

The importance of interaction: reclaiming social interaction

As stated earlier, social interaction is what makes the social world go round. It constitutes virtually the whole of human activity. The work of Goffman (1968, 1969, 1972, 1981) has been particularly influential in this area. Goffman argues that social interaction comprises not only behaviour in public places, social encounters, conversations, assaults and so on but also television and radio broadcasts and talking to oneself (1981).

It is Goffman's work on the experience of spoiled identity that is of most interest to disability studies. In *Stigma* social interaction is premised on the notion that 'Society establishes the means of categorising persons and the complement of attributes felt to be ordinary and natural for members of each of these categories' (Goffman 1968, p. 11). A person's appearance allows us to place him or her into a category, allocating them what Goffman termed a 'social identity'. The categorisation system, for Goffman, exists outside of these encounters, and is applied unreflectively (p. 12). Similarly the concept of 'normality' is assumed. People with a visible physical impairment are, according to Goffman, discredited, unable to achieve full 'humanness'. So he writes: 'By definition, of course we believe that a person with a stigma is not quite human' (p. 15) and people who are discredited face discrimination which reduces their life chances. This unequal treatment is, Goffman believes, justified by other, non-discredited people, through the creation of a 'stigma theory', an ideology which permits such treatment of the discredited on the grounds of their stigma.

Through interactions, 'shared vocabularies of body idiom' (1968, p. 35) emerge. These vocabularies allow us to grade individuals, providing us with hierarchies according to unspecified categories. Any violations of these situational norms are treated as signs of instability, body management being central to social interaction. Giddens (1991), drawing on Goffman and Garfinkel, applies similar criteria in his analysis of the body and identity. Not only can disabled people's bodies appear threatening, but by acting in an unpredictable manner, for example spasticity, they operate outside of any 'shared vocabularies of body idiom'. An impaired body can disrupt the social hierarchy, disabled people are thus seen as dependent.

Further, as Lois Keith (1996) argues, social interactions between disabled and non-disabled people are characterised by confusion and problem. She draws on the writings of Murphy, who argues:

> The disabled person must make an extra effort to establish his status as an autonomous, worthy individual but the reaction of the other party may totally undercut these pretensions through some thoughtless act or omission. Even if the able bodied person is making a conscious attempt to pay deference to the disabled party, he must struggle against the underlying ambiguity of the encounter, the lack of clear cultural guidelines on how to behave and perhaps his own sense of revulsion.
>
> (1987, p. 103)

She suggests that all rules become altered in the interaction between disabled and non-disabled people.

For people with a physical impairment, stigma is, in Goffman's formulation, embodied. The stigmata are also recognised by the stigmatised, who share the same sense of normality as the undefined normals (Goffman 1968, pp. 17–18). Impaired people are thus cast in the position of outsider, placed on the margins of society by virtue of their impairment. It is this embodiment of stigma that is problematic in this analysis. Goffman is not interested in causes, he brackets any reference to the creation of these categories and while his work is more than mere description it is free from value judgements around how individuals interact with those he classifies as stigmatised. The concept of stigma, and its embodiment on the stigmatised ignores the broader roles of cultural representation which render disabled people 'other'. If the concept of stigma were to be recast around the concept of prejudice a far more powerful analysis could be achieved, in that the blame for such prejudice would fall squarely on the shoulders of the 'normal'. It may be argued that he is only interested in spoiled interaction as a means to cast light on 'normal' interaction. However, as Goffman himself argues (1968), we all have some stigma of our own, a point echoed in the writings of Bauman (1996).

Goffman has been widely criticised for his concentration on the micro and his omission of socio-economic power and inequality. His work has been criticised by many within disability studies; for example Finkelstein (1981) accuses him of individualising the issue and Oliver (1990), of an over-reliance on psychological models and secondary sources. Oliver concludes:

> ... while stigma may be an appropriate metaphor for describing what happens to individual disabled people in social interactions, it is unable to explain why this stigmatisation occurs or to incorporate collective rather than personal responses to stigma. (1990, p. 66)

However, towards the end of *Stigma* Goffman clearly recognises that these criticisms could be made of his work when he argues:

> Sociologically, the central issue concerning these groups [the stigmatised] is their place in the social structure; the contingencies these persons encounter in face-to-face interaction is only part of the problem, and something that cannot itself be fully understood without reference to the history, the political development and the current policies of the group. (Goffman 1968, p. 151)

Goffman's work provides, however, a crucial amendment to the social model theorists. By tackling the issue of presentational non-conformity and exploring the dominating effects that it can have on social interaction, he challenges the assumption implicit in their approach, demonstrating that there is more to disablement than material, institutional or statutory barriers (Shakespeare 1994a). It also clearly repositions the problem of impairment from the body to the social, in that it is the social that creates the stigma.

Prejudice

As a consequence of the prevailing focus of disability studies and its emphasis on the material, we have a wide range of literature documenting the discrimination that disabled people face in the workplace, in health services and in education (see for example Barnes' *Disabled People in Britain and Discrimination* 1991). However, with the exception of the collection edited by Hunt in 1966, there has been little exploration of the cultural representation of disabled people in the UK and the prejudice that this produces for disabled people. Oliver, as Shakespeare (1994b) points out, barely mentions cultural issues in either of his two major works on disablement. Morris (1991) and Keith (1996) have addressed this issue from an anecdotal rather than sociological perspective. Shakespeare (1994b) has examined this from a theoretical angle. By drawing on the work of Mary Douglas, Victor Turner and Simone de Beauvoir, he argues that disabled people remind non-disabled people of their own mortality and morbidity and as such are scapegoated, becoming what Heavey (1991) has called 'dustbins for disavowal'. This chapter adopts an empirical approach on exploring how disabled people perceive the prejudice they experience.

The data presented are drawn from interviews with 28 disabled people. The informants were all volunteers recruited through housing associations, sports clubs and organisations of and for disabled people. Each person was interviewed twice over a six-month period; analysis was carried out using the standard protocols for qualitative analysis (Lofland and Lofland 1995). All the informants have been given pseudonyms and their identity has been further protected by the removal of any non-essential information that may be used to identify them.

The daily experience of oppression

All the participants described how, in their everyday lives, they were the subject of oppression or oppressive practices. Although violence was rare, three of the informants described how they had been attacked in the street. For example Sheila commented:

> I was out with some friends from work the other week. I don't get as much slagging as I used to – it's younger people. But if I do I just give them an earful back. But I was walking down Lothian Road in the early hours of the morning there was a guy on the outside of the pavement and I was on the inside of the pavement, and I saw what he was going to do, he came from the outside of the pavement carrying his boxes of pizza straight in and kicked the crutch away. It's ignorance. He came from the outside of the pavement in, I could see him – smash, kick.

Arnie had also been the subject of a violent attack, but refused to talk about it, it was he said 'too personal'. Anne talked about how she often, especially late at night had to put up with comments about the way that she walks:

> **NW:** Have people victimised you for being disabled?
>
> **Anne:** Em, it can, right, it can happen in the street. Like a couple of Sundays ago ... 'And what are you walking ...' no, 'You cannae walk ...' This guy was rolling down the window – I was at Haymarket end, going to see my friend, she wasn't in, right – and he rolled it down and said, 'Oh, you cannae walk right.' A complete stranger!

One of the participants had been the victim of sexual abuse, and whilst it cannot be argued that she was abused because she was disabled, her abuser was in a position of power over her, and able to use this power to allow him to both ensure her silence and her future cooperation. In this way he was able to regularly rape this woman, over a period of three years.

These attacks are the consequence of both powerlessness and violence. As Connell (1987, p. 107) argues, with respect to rape, violence should not be viewed as a means of deviation from the social order, but as a means of reinforcing it. Attacks such as these are very difficult, and at times impossible, for individuals to resist. Resistance at the time of the assault may antagonise the assailant and further the aggression (Carter *et al.* 1988). While the feminist movement has made violence against women visible (Kelly 1988), violence against disabled people has tended to be unreported (Shakespeare *et al.* 1996). Disabled people who have been abused in such a way should not be seen as victims but as 'actively engaged in a struggle to cope with the consequences of abuse' (Kelly 1988, p. 159). The focus is then on the way that individuals cope with, resist and survive without damaging their subjectivity. In the example of Sheila above, when the abuse was verbal she felt able to respond, resisting the assault, yet when the attack became physical she was unable to do so. Resistance can only be achieved by dismissing the assault as the consequence of 'ignorance'. This is discussed later. Similarly with Arnie: the attack was something that he refused to discuss, a coping strategy that Kelly (1988) sees as an adaptive process to facilitate survival.

Other forms of oppression were also widespread. This took many forms, the most common of which was what they nearly all described as 'Does she (or he) take sugar?' In this example the disabled person is ignored, and made invisible. As Arnie says:

> It's more they look at you and they tend to patronise you, sort of pat you on the head, and if you're with somebody, ask, 'Does Johnny take sugar in his tea or coffee?' instead of asking the person.

This occurred on an almost daily basis to most of the participants. Many of the participants described how they were often assumed to have a learning difficulty because they had a physical impairment, a relationship that they rejected and found offensive. Disabled people are thus marginalised, excluded from the mainstream of social interaction, or have to overcome barriers to get there and to participate.

In other examples the disabled person is depersonalised, treated as if not only are they not there, but also as if they have no feelings, so Deirdre says:

> The other day I was being pushed by a friend and somebody came up and said to him 'Doing your good deed for the day are you?'. I was too shocked to say anything.

Some of the participants also described how non-disabled people seemed to view them as incapable of doing things on their own, as being unable to manage their own lives. So Keiron says:

I mean myself and my dad we used to get this all the time, and I remember once being in Glasgow and there was a crowd of people that went to the garden festival there, and there was lady of about 60, and I was just sitting on the park bench and my dad was there and she said, 'What home are you from?' because she thought the people we were with were all institutionalised, you see. And my dad said, 'Nobody's from any home, we're just a group of people out for a day'. And then she's saying, my dad was telling her some of the things that we did in the group and she looked almost amazed, it was this great big shock.

Oppression as patronage and the denial of agency

Many of the participants described how they were treated as children. For example Leslie, describing her relationship with her district nurse, says:

She's got one of these cheery dispositions and she tries very hard to be on a level with me but it still comes through this kind of 'You're a busy girl, aren't you, what are you doing today, oh you're working today, you're a busy girl'. Or she brings a student in and she'll say, 'This young lady, she's very busy, aren't you Lesley?' And I just think, 'Fuck off!'

Resistance in this example is indirect, unspoken, but still present. In any relationship with health professionals, resistance is difficult. Not only do they have medical dominance over the individual, but with disabled people the relationship is more intense, and at times more controlling. Stewart talked about how he had to have medical tests to travel by plane, something that he felt that he himself should be able to decide:

Stewart: I think it is unnecessary to do it because I know what I want in my own life and take the correct equipment with me that I require and I think it is again an infringement on my ability to travel.
NW: Right.
Stewart: I know what I can do.
NW: You don't think it should be up to the medical profession?
Stewart: I don't think so, I don't think we should have to turn to them and say look, is it OK to travel? I think I should be able to travel by myself.

By demanding such tests, his agency is removed and any notion that he may have knowledge of how to deal with his impairment is challenged. This serves to remind him that not only is he impaired, but also that major decisions about his life can be taken out of his control. This removal of control became particularly evident when dealing with professions allied to medicine, particularly the occupational therapist. Marion, when talking about her new bathroom and kitchen that were being installed at the time of my second visit, described how her views on any adaptations had been ignored by the occupational therapist. The therapist insisted on installing a new toilet of a different height to the previous one, a height that Marion found difficult to transfer to. Even though Marion fell off the toilet a number of times the therapist refused to accept her point of view and eventually Marion herself had to pay to have a new toilet fitted. As a result of this action, the therapist threatened to withhold payment for the rest of the work, saying that she felt that the new arrangements were unsafe. As she says:

> I feel that you are hitting your head off a brick wall all the time and getting nowhere.

Nearly all the informants talked about occurrences such as these, illustrating the way that control is removed from the individual. Despite living with their impairments, and learning how best to adapt things around them, their views were seldom listened to. They were powerless, and unless, like Marion, they have the financial capacity to rectify the problems created by others, they must live with the consequences.

Some informants also talked about how, whenever they had a medical problem members of the health professions rarely listened to them and tended to locate any health problem that they had in their pre-existing impairment. As Bob described a recent trip to the hospital and his GP following an accident:

> **Bob:** My GP, for example, I walk in and he says 'How is your leg?' 'Still here'. 'How is this, fine' 'Why are you here?' 'I just happened to crack my knee cap'. He was looking at my bad leg so I said 'Not that one, my good one'. 'How did you fall?' 'Like anybody else'. You know, I mean, to me they're silly questions but I suppose they're not. And I start firing silly answers back and I think now he realises that I tell him what is wrong with me. It's the same in hospital. I was on a trolley, the doctor came in and said 'Knee caps', I said 'No, just one'. 'It says knee caps here'. I said,

'I don't care what's on my sheet, it is knee cap one, left. That is the right one, that is the left one.' It took him about five minutes for me to get him to realise he has to ask me the questions and I would answer him sensibly. He was going to 'ok' what was on the sheet. The sheet can only tell you so much, the patient can tell you a lot more.

NW: So they don't really listen to you?

Bob: They treat you like a piece of meat. They know I am a wheelchair user. That is why you are in a wheelchair but if you have a cut finger, sore head, a patch over your left eye but they still see the wheelchair.

What this shows and what became evident throughout the interviews was how sophisticated the informants were in their use of, and relationship with, health professionals. When dealing with their GP or regular consultant many had managed to negotiate a relationship in which they had taken charge and laid down the boundaries. As Stella says:

If I think something needs treating, I will discuss it with my GP and I'll ask her for a range of options. If I'm seeing a specialist, as I do occasionally, I will make sure that – well most of my consultants now know me enough to talk to me at a fairly sophisticated level – I just need to know all the information that's going. I haven't found that to be the case across the board. When you establish a relationship with a health professional, then you can work on that. There are several instances I can quote, however, where my experience of health professionals is very negative.

In this way some of the informants were able to resist domination by the health professional, challenging the image of themselves as powerless and reclaiming agency. However, this was usually only achieved through prolonged contact

Many of the informants had taken part in 'training' of health service professionals. Whilst they were unsure of the roles that the professionals expected them to take, they were very sure of their own reasons for taking part. John described how he went to the local medical school to tell the students how to treat him and people like him, to look beyond his impairment, to 'tell it like it really is'. That if he was ill, they were not to look to his impairment first but to look at him as a whole. These are similar actions to those of the Boston Women's Health Co-operative in

America (Frank 1995). By challenging the way that professionals learnt about disability, they felt that they could alter the way that they, and others like them, would be treated in the future.

Oppression as the product of charity

The participants talked about how they were often patronised and treated as people who should be pitied, the object of charity. Javid described how, when he was sitting waiting for a taxi outside the theatre with his hat on his knees, a coach load of tourists pulled up and as they filed past him put money in his hat. Even when he told them he didn't want their money they carried on giving it to him. He had to move back inside the theatre. This image of a disabled person as one in need of charity was, many of the informants felt, the product of the media. As Keiron argues:

> When I was growing up, the only images you saw of disabled people were like a wee five-minute piece on like *Blue Peter* or something where they'd say, 'This year's special appeal, for a minibus', or whatever, this type of thing. Or you'd maybe see, I don't know, a play and I think a lot of the images, I can't stand things like Esther Rantzen programmes, you know, *Hearts of Gold* and all that, all this type of stuff because to that is very 'deserving cripples'. Yeah, it's all, 'Does a lot charity', and it's incredibly irritating. I think how people are presented, it's like if they said, for example, if they said we'll portray black people so we'll only show bits of *Gone With The Wind*, everybody's a slave and that, everybody's stereotyped.

The media were felt to be at the root of many of the ideas about disability that were prevalent in society. Disabled people were portrayed, according to the informants as 'less than average,' as 'negative,' as 'dependent' and as 'people to be pitied'. Many commented on the fact that disabled people were rarely seen outside of stereotypical settings; as Marion says:

> **Marion:** Well they're not on the television enough, and if they are on the television, it's usually a very condescending story line that's used round about them.

> **NW:** Such as what, what do you mean...?
>
> **Marion:** Well, they're the 'too poor person', you know, how can I put it, you feel that the people who are running the programmes have put them in just as a token representation, not for the main reason of why they should be in. Does that sound right? They're always given a negative image.

This was something that many felt was damaging to them, not directly as individuals watching the television, but as they negotiated their way through life. It affected the way that other, non-disabled, people communicated with them and saw them. Many talked about the rare examples in the media where they were presented in a better light and how this cheered them. The older participants talked fondly of *Crossroads* and *Ironsides* whilst the younger tended to focus on the few examples in more recent programmes. For example Anne:

> **Anne:** Yeah, yeah, nobody would... but I have to praise, actually, Grange Hill for portraying a disabled person. I thought that was great. Have you watched Grange Hill?
>
> **NW:** No, I've not.
>
> **Anne:** There was a girl with CP, well, I'd say a lot worse than me. And I thought, good on you, because these workmen said, 'You've been a bit young to go to the pub!' And this lassie who was non-disabled 'em, she says, 'em, wait a minute till I get this right... 'Haven't you met somebody with CP before?' And I was going, cheering at the telly. 'Cos the image they had got that...

Becoming the centre of attention

Many of the informants talked about how they were often made the centre of unasked-for attention, treated as if having an impairment makes it permissible for other people to ask them deeply personal questions, which are usually related to their impairment, such as 'What is wrong with you, why are you in that chair?' and so on. This was not always seen as offensive, for example many of the participants felt that it was only natural that children should be inquisitive, 'Wondering what that big lady's doing in a "pushchair"' as Caroline puts it. However, it was the reaction of the children's parents that many found upsetting, by pulling their children away, telling them not to stare and so on, implying that they were not to be looked at, that they were other, further making them invisible and increasing their marginalisation. Marks (1997) has likened this to what Hall (1990) cites as the question most frequently asked of migrants: 'Why are you here?' and 'When are you going back home?' (Hall 1990, p. 44). She argues that by asking questions about an individual's impairment, the very existence of disabled people is presented as a problem. However, it may also be argued that non-disabled people are asking such questions in an attempt to create a barrier between themselves and disabled people, not only to try and ensure that are they not seen as disabled, but also to reduce the possibility that they themselves are at risk of becoming disabled (see Crawford 1994).

For many of the participants, when they were asked what was wrong with them, or why they were in a chair it was seen as an opportunity to put their side of the story, to explain their situation and to challenge other people's perceptions of them. So Jane says:

> **Jane:** You know, if you're out, say, and a child's looking at you and the mother'll drag them away, 'Don't be rude, you don't look at them like that'. But maybe the child just wants to say, 'Why are you in that, what's wrong with you? Why can't you walk?'
>
> **NW:** And you're quite happy to answer those sorts of questions?
>
> **Jane:** Yes. When my daughter first went to school she used to say, 'Don't take me to school, you dress like a tramp'. And this really hurt me. But that wasn't the problem, it was the remarks being made to her because her mum was in a wheelchair. So I asked the teacher at school if I could go over and talk to the children and just explain to them, and then they were totally different. They used to come and offer to help you and, do you want your dog walked, or do you want messages or things. It all boils down to just ignorance.

Whilst Jane did not mind responding to the children's questions, many respondents resented questions about how impairments were acquired because these reproduced the stereotypical presentations of disabled people in the media. If, as often happens in the media, disabled people are only seen in situations in which they are being asked to describe their impairments and the medical consequences of these impairments, it is hardly surprising that on meeting disabled people, non-disabled people feel able to adopt a similar manner to that of the media. The presentation of disabled people in the media extends the medical gaze beyond the clinic.

This invasion of other people's lives extended beyond asking about the impairment. Disabled people believed they were seen as being incapable and untrustworthy, as Joyce describes:

> Because it comes up time and time again. And I'll tell you one strange thing that happened. I took the bairns out to the pictures and it was a Saturday afternoon. I paid for the tickets and got them an ice-cream and somebody said to me 'Should you be out with the kids on your own?'.

Not only are they seen as being incapable of looking after their own bodies and lives, but also of being unable to look after others.

Attention is also increased by physical barriers, by steps or heavy doors. Many talked about how slopes or curbs made non-disabled people feel that they should step in and help, further creating the image that disabled people are dependent on help. This presented the informants with a dilemma. If it was a situation which they could manage they often felt patronised when people did step in, but, as Jose points out, it is difficult to know if you might need help in the future:

> But even when they are condescending you say, 'Thank you very much but I'll manage. It was very kind of you'. Because you never know when there'll come a day when you will need somebody to help you.

Engaging with non-disabled people

Many of the participants talked about the way that non-disabled people had difficulty in, or were embarrassed by, or scared of, talking to them. As Deirdre noted:

> **Deirdre:** ...they have backed off because I have spoken and the person with me hasn't, it is almost to say 'it can talk, it talked to me'.
>
> **NW:** Do you think you scare people?
>
> **Deirdre:** Well, I think the wheelchair scares them.
>
> **NW:** Why?

> **Deirdre:** As I said before, they see the chair before me so it might scare people that I have actually got a voice and I can speak for myself because a lot of people don't see disabled people like that.

This need to educate non-disabled people was something that came up throughout all the interviews. As this work was funded by the Health Education Board for Scotland, a section on health education was included in the interviews. A number of the informants felt that one of the roles of health education should be to challenge the way that non-disabled people view disability. As Jane argues:

> **Jane:** I think there should be more done with changing attitudes and things.
>
> **NW:** Changing attitudes?
>
> **Jane:** Yes, yes. There is not enough about disability at school or anything. I mean I never got taught anything at school.

The issue of segregated education was also seen as being at the root of what was termed the ignorance of non-disabled people. Deirdre described how, after going through segregated primary and secondary education and then moving on to a segregated residential college for four years post school, she knew little about life outside of institutions. This was brought home to her when she moved into mainstream further education:

> **Deirdre:** It took me a long time because I went on a course in —, it was for able-bodied, you know, and I was the only disabled person on it. And that was difficult because they had their own wee cliques and stuff, I wasn't involved in them for a long time.
>
> **NW:** Do you think that's because they didn't want to know you ?
>
> **Deirdre:** They didn't know how to speak to me.

She went on further to describe them as ignorant.

● Oppression as ignorance

The notion of 'ignorance' was used by almost all the informants to defend the comments of non-disabled people, as if they didn't really mean what they were saying because they didn't really understand what it was to be disabled. For example when I asked Javid how he felt about the people who had treated him like they did outside the theatre, he replied 'They're just ignorant, they don't understand. It's just down to ignorance'. As Joyce argued:

> How can I put it? I don't know whether you have seen it, but there was an advert on the telly recently about pouring the kettle with your feet and that. I was at the dentist in Duncan Street and on the video in the waiting-room – they have things like they have in the doctors' surgery – and there was a couple of able-bodied in the waiting-room and I was just watching this room ... and they said ... 'Isn't that marvellous?' and I thought to myself 'What's marvellous about that? She's just doing day-to-day things like everybody else would.' So I said to them, I turned round to them 'I'm sorry but I couldn't help hearing you'. I said 'Why do you think it is so marvellous?' And they gave me a definition of it which was quite good. 'I have never come across a person with that disability. If only doctors and that told you more about certain conditions, they would be interested'. So then I thought 'That's a good answer, it was an honest one from them and I thought, you know, perhaps we do need to do that'.

This idea of prejudice as a result of ignorance was, in many accounts, supported by the informants' experiences with friends. Many argued that on first meeting them they could, by the force of their own personality, persuade non-disabled people that they were 'normal'. Jane put this eloquently:

> Well you've got to prove to them that you're a woman first and you're disabled second. You're a human being.

Conclusion

Oliver (1996) has suggested that a focus on the prejudice that disabled people experience implies a return to an individualistic model of disability. It can further be argued that an exploration of the concept of prejudice implies an analysis that is rooted in psychology, suggesting a similarity to other phobias. It must be remembered that the prejudice faced by disabled people and the second class status ascribed to them, is the result of oppression. As Kitzinger (1987) argues, in relation to homophobia, there is a danger that a focus on prejudice can result in an analysis of 'personal pathology of specific individuals who deviate from the supposedly egalitarian norms of society, thus obscuring analysis of our oppression as a political problem rooted in social institutions and organisations' (p. 154). It runs the risk of individualising the problem (Plummer 1981).

However, as argued earlier, any quest to understand and challenge the oppression faced by disabled people can only benefit from an analysis of the ways in which prejudice is reproduced. This prejudice is produced in particular life-worlds and social contexts and such analysis allows for its contextualisation and examination of the apparatuses of society that serve to create the prejudice and constrain people's life chances. Through this a picture of how the cultural representation of disabled people is mobilised and reinforced and oppresses disabled people, from the perspective of disabled people, can emerge. It is also possible to see how in turn this might be curbed or dissipated. As Keith argues 'an analysis of these apparently minor, but actually very significant events in the lives of disabled people, what they mean and what effects they have on us, is part of the political progress disabled people are making' (1996, p. 75).

To turn this into a political strategy, then, requires a means by which this hurt engendered by private experiences of injury is channelled into political actions that accord with the political aspirations of the disabled people's movement. A language needs to be developed which allows for the forming of a model of disablement through which these feelings of hurt can be seen not as individual assaults, but as part of a systematic attack which can be shown to be typical for disabled people as a whole. The social model, with its denial of the importance of experience and its emphasis on material relations, fails in this in many ways. Disablement is not solely, at an individual level, perceived to be an attack on material opportunities. Disabled people are not only competing for scarce goods in a market place. Rather, disablement is felt as the outcome of the withholding of social and cultural recognition, and it is this that should form the basis of the social struggle.

The work of the German political theorist Axel Honneth might be useful here. Honneth (1995) argues that it is important to reconcile the individual as well as the collective dimensions of political struggles. For him, self-confidence, self-respect and self-esteem provide the possibility of identity formation. This works at three levels: relationships, legal rights and solidarity. In relation to solidarity, Honneth is not referring merely to solidarity within groups, but, importantly, between groups. Through relationships, self-confidence emerges; through rights, a sense of personal dignity emerges; and through solidarity, self esteem grows. Denial of relationships can result in a loss of physical integrity, denial of self-respect, social integrity, and denial of self-esteem can damage honour and dignity. It is a need for recognition that drives minority communities to mobilise for change and it is the negative emotional reactions that result from the experiences of being denied recognition that form the motivational basis for social struggle. He cites the work of the Marxist historian E.P. Thompson (1963), who suggests that social rebellion requires more than economic hardship. It requires a violation of the accepted moral consensus, a denial of what are felt to be the moral expectations of people within that community, which means recognition.

While it is true that disablism is deeply embedded in contemporary society and that disabling societal macro-structures need to be analysed and challenged, by focusing on the denial of recognition a more experiential strategy can be achieved. Disabling social relations are everywhere, they are part of disabled people's everyday life and a movement founded on such is more likely to find accord with disabled people. The challenges that many of the informants made when they felt that recognition was denied add weight to this argument. Disabled people, everyday, confront disablism. What is needed, if the movement is to become more relevant to disabled people, is a recognition of the importance of cultural equality and political recognition.

References

Barnes, C. (1991) *Disabled people in Britain and discrimination*, Hurst and Co, London.

Bauman, Z. (1996) 'From pilgrim to tourist: or a short history of identity' in Halls and du Gay, P. (eds) *Questions of Cultural Identity*, Sage, London.

Bourdieu, P. (1998) *Practical Reason*, Polity Press, Cambridge.

Connell, R. (1987) *Gender and Power*, Polity Press, Cambridge.

Carter, D., Prentky, R. and Burgess, A. (1988) 'Victims: Lessons learned for responses to sexual violence' in Ressler, R., Burgess, A. and Douglas, J. (eds) *Sexual Homicides: patterns and motives*, Lexington Books, Lexington, MA.

Crawford, R. (1994) 'The boundaries of the self and the unhealthy other: Reflections on health, culture and AIDS', *Social Sciences and Medicine*, **38**, pp. 1347–1365.

Elias, N. (1994) *The Civilising Process*, Blackwell, Oxford.

Finkelstein, V. (1981) 'To deny or not to deny disability' in Brechin, A., Liddiard, P. and Swain, J. (eds) *Handicap in a social world*, Hodder and Stoughton, Milton Keynes.

Frank, A. (1995) *The wounded story teller: Body, illness and ethics*, University of Chicago Press, London.

Giddens, A. (1991) *Modernity and Self Identity*, Polity Press, Cambridge.

Goffman, E. (1968) *Stigma*, Pelican, Harmondsworth.

Goffman, E. (1969) *The Presentation of the Self in Everyday Life*, Allan Lane, London.

Goffman, E. (1972) *Relations in Public*, Harper Colophon Books, London.

Goffman, E. (1979) *Gender Advertisements*, Macmillan, Basingstoke.

Goffman, E. (1981) *Forms of Talk*, Blackwell, Cambridge.

Hall, S. (1990) 'Cultural Identity and Diaspora' in Rutherford, J. (ed.) *Identity: Community, Culture, Difference*, Lawrence and Wishart, London.

Hevey, D. (1992) *The Creatures Time Forgot: Photography and Disability Imagery*, Routledge, London.

Honneth, A. (1995) *The Struggle for Recognition: The Moral Grammar of Social Conflicts*, Polity Press, Cambridge.

Hunt, P. (ed.) (1998) *Stigma: The experience of disability*, Chapman, London.

Keith, L. (1996) 'Encounters with Strangers' in Morris, J. (ed.) *Encounters with strangers*, The Women's Press, London.

Kelly, L. (1988) *Surviving Sexual Violence Polity*, Cambridge University Press, Cambridge.

Kitzinger, C. (1987) *The social construction of lesbianism*, Sage, London.

Lemert, C. (1997) *Postmodernism is not what you think*, Blackwell, Oxford.

Lofland, J. and Lofland, L. (1995) *Analysing social settings*, 3rd edn, Wadsworth, California.

Marks, D. (1997) 'Disability and Cultural Citizenship', paper presented at *Disability Studies Seminar*, Edinburgh.

Morris, J. (1991) *Pride Against Prejudice*, The Women's Press, London.

Murphy, R. (1987) *The Body Silent*, Henry Holt, New York.

Oliver, M. (1990) *The Politics of Disablement*, Macmillan, Basingstoke.

Oliver, M. (1996) *Understanding disability: From theory to practice*, Macmillan, Basingstoke.

Plummer, K. (1981) *The Making of the Modern Homosexual*, Barnes and Noble, Totowa, NJ.

Shakespeare, T. (1994a) Unpublished D.Phil. thesis, University of Cambridge.

Shakespeare, T. (1994b) 'Cultural representation of disabled people: Dustbins for disavowal', *Disability Handicap and Society*, 8(3), pp. 249–264.

Shakespeare, T., Gillespie-Sells, K. and Davies, D. (1996) *The Sexual Politics of Disability: untold desires*, Cassell, London.

Thompson, E.P. (1963) *The Making of the English Working Class*, Gollancz, London.

CHAPTER 4

'It's like your hair going grey', or is it?: impairment, disability and the habitus of old age

Mark Priestley

Introduction

This chapter highlights some important similarities and differences in the cultural construction of old age and disability. The first part of the chapter outlines some of the key approaches to thinking about disability and old age, in terms of structure, culture, the ageing body and identity. The second part highlights some of the ways in which those working with older disabled people construct and think about disability and old age. The data used to illustrate this account are taken from research involving local voluntary sector organisations working with, and representing the interests of, older people. The chapter concludes with a discussion of the relationship between impairment, disability and the habitus of old age, including the implications for identity maintenance in old age, within the context of late modernity.

Thinking about disability and old age

The argument presented in this chapter is based on an assumption that there are important commonalities in the cultural construction of old age and disability, and that there are also similarities in the way that older people and disabled people have been represented through culture. The various contributions to this volume provide a detailed analysis of the way in which disability is produced and maintained through identity and culture and, with this in mind, it is useful to focus first on the construction of old age.

There are many ways of thinking about old age, and about the meaning of becoming an older person. Old age has been constructed in a number of ways, and it is important to review some of the most important approaches in order to understand how culture and identity are embedded within, and expressed through, for example, macro-social structures and the ageing body.

First, there is a sense in which the ageing process remains fundamentally a biological one. After all, the human body in its biological sense is a finite entity, and many of our cultural understandings of old age, and the consequent identities of older people, are grounded in our perceptions about the frailty of the physical body resulting from ageing processes. There is much similarity here with the biological determinism of medical models of disability. Yet the body is not simply biological. It is also constructed through cultural meanings and disciplined through discourse (Corker 2001; Corker and French 1999; Katz 1996). Just as the impaired body has often come to signify disability so the ageing body has often come to signify what we understand as old age. Understanding the role of discourse is important because representations of disability and old age that rely on perceptions of the physical frailty of the human body frequently serve to legitimise the medicalised surveillance and discipline of older and disabled people's real lives. This theme is explored later in discussing the relationship between perceptions of impairment and the ageing body.

Second, conflict theories have been useful in offering an explanation of old age as structural dependency, created through the social relations of production under capitalism, and sustained through older people's unequal access to the economic products of capital accumulation. In particular, such approaches have emphasised how an administrative or bureaucratic category of older people was created with the introduction of formal retirement from labour force participation within Western industrialised economies (Minkler and Estes 1991; Phillipson 1982). Such an explanation has much in common with social model theories of disability, particularly as articulated by writers such as Oliver (1990) or Finkelstein (1991).

However, the emphasis within conflict theory on the structural location of generational conflict does not fully explain the cultural meanings that we attribute to old age, which tend to be more situated and contextual. Consequently, a third general approach is to view old age in terms of the identities of older people, for example in the process of 'becoming older'. Here, the emphasis has been to concentrate primarily on the maintenance of individual identities in their biographical context over the life course (e.g. Thompson, Itzin and Abendstern 1990). How people construct their identities, and the narratives that they use to do this, are the results of complicated social and reflexive processes. These personal constructions and narratives are important in understanding old-age identities. However, in this chapter the emphasis is on the constructions of old age used by others (and specifically by those working with and for older people in voluntary organsiations).

Both older people and disabled people, of all ages, have been constructed as negative categories in opposition to an idealised notion of adulthood. Within this idealised view, adults have been viewed as occupying independent and autonomous roles that contribute to production and reproduction. These roles have of course been highly gendered within the context of modernity. For example, our idealised construction of male adult roles has centred on the ability to perform an autonomous role as worker, within the social relations of capitalist production, and as breadwinner, within the private sphere of domestic patriarchy. Conversely, the cultural construction of women within the same context has tended to emphasise both the resilience and nurturing autonomy of motherhood and a simultaneous dependency upon men (both in the public and private domain).

These traditional and modernist discourses of adulthood have promoted values such as the work ethic, youth, productivity and progress, thereby devaluing the position of older people in society. However, the emergence of a more consumerist culture has led some to contend that the cultural values of consumption have begun to outweigh values based on production. Within the context of late modernity, participation, citizenship and personhood are increasingly measured with reference to cultural consumption rather than production, and such conclusions have a strong resonance for a generation of retired people with more access to the resources needed in order to consume and to enjoy leisure participation (Laslett 1989). So, within a context of late modernity, the advent of the 'Third Age' has been seen to have more in common with constructions of adulthood than with the presumed structural dependency and physical decline of traditional ageing.

Thus, while the phase of active adulthood expands to embrace many more seniors, stronger taboos form around those in poverty, those whose pastimes lack positive cultural resonances, and those suffering from disability (sic) and diseases such as Alzheimer's.   (Blaikie 1999)

To summarise: individually, it is important to be able to think about old age in terms of the ageing body, both biologically and as that body is produced through participation in the social relations of production and reproduction. It is also possible to think about old age in terms of individual biography and identity, either as disruption or as consistency in personal narratives of later life. Collectively, old age may be viewed as a structural or an administrative category deployed to control changing labour supply, and maintained through disciplining discourses. It may equally be viewed as a cultural identity category, constructed and situated in relation to other generational categories (such as adulthood or childhood). As Blaikie concludes:

> To the extent that it acts as an organising principle, ageing may be understood either by reference to perspectives that emphasise structural organisation of society ... (or) interpretive, processual theories, concerned with individuals and the roles of meanings.   (Blaikie 1999)

Clearly, there are many parallels here with the way in which we think about and construct disability. As I have argued elsewhere, there are in fact many significant similarities in the way that generational categories and categories of disability have been culturally constructed and socially produced (Priestley 2000; Priestley 2001). In order to look at how such concepts work in practice it is helpful to draw on some examples.

Talking about older disabled people

The following examples are drawn from interviews with key informants working in local voluntary organisations that either provide services to, or represent, older people. The purpose of the research project was to investigate the potential for greater political alliance in collaboration between organisations of older people and organisations of disabled people. We were interested in the claims made on behalf of old and disabled people and in the voices representing those claims. More details about these aspects of the research are included in other publications arising from the project (Priestley 2002; Priestley and Rabiee 2001). Here the discussion focuses on the way in which our informants talked about the older people they claimed to represent, and what this can tell us about the cultural construction of old age and disability.

The majority of disabled people in Britain are over retirement age and all of the 21 organisations we visited were working with older people who had impairments. Yet few chose to represent their interests in terms of disability issues or identities (with the exception of some disability organisations). In our discussions we became aware of a high degree of cognitive dissonance in the accounts of our interviewees. For example, on the one hand they would argue that there are 'no disabled people here', while on the other hand admitting that, 'they're all disabled in some way'. The following examples give a flavour of the complexity of these accounts.

Preoccupations with the body and physical function

One of our key research interests was to examine the way in which organisations working with older people think about and construct old age and disability. We looked at the way they defined their constituency and at the way they talked about disability in relation to old age. In particular, we sought to draw out some of the language and discourses used to explain relationships between impairment, disability, and old age (Ylanne-McEwen 1999). An important strand in this analysis was to identify the ways in which older people's organisations included or excluded people with impairments in defining the older people they sought to represent.

The legitimacy of medical models of disability has been premised upon the assumption that the disadvantage experienced by disabled people is largely a product of the imperfect body (Dutton 1996). Thus, the traditional cultural construction of disability has drawn disproportionately upon the physicality of certain kinds of impairment, while the medicalisation of disability has been founded upon a scaling of bodies against physical norms in order to create disciplinary categories of deviation. It was not surprising then to find in our interviews that perceptions of the transition to both old age and disability were often characterised by a preoccupation with certain kinds of physical impairment (predominantly visible mobility impairments).

In some cases, the term disability was used only to describe older people with visible physical impairments. For example:

> I don't like to label people. I wouldn't label somebody as having it unless it's physical and you cannot avoid, and the person has got the appearance of whatever ... when you label people disabled, you put them in that category that makes other people see them different.

In this sense, only significant physical mobility impairments were sometimes perceived as 'real disability'. Thus, 'Most of them . . . have a disability of some kind . . . No-one comes in calliper or in a wheelchair. Nobody is as bad as that. They come with sticks . . .' (the distinction of impairments regarded as 'normal' in old age is addressed later). More constructivist theorising about old age has tended to obscure the physical body, yet we found that the appearance and trappings of the impaired body were very important in how people thought about disability in old age.

Similarly, Oberg (1996) draws attention to the paradoxical 'absence of the body' from social gerontology (paradoxical because of the prevalence of bodily discourse in popular cultural constructions of old age and older people). However, contemporary cultural and social theorists have become more interested in thinking about the ageing body in terms of impairment or 'limiting illness' (Gilleard and Higgs 1998). There are evident parallels here with attempts to reintroduce the body and impairment into discussions of disability identity within a social model (e.g. Hughes and Paterson 1997).

In our research the onset of old age was often associated explicitly with the onset of impairment. This association between impairment and old age was generally explained in relation to physical functioning, for example, with reference to people being unable to do 'something that you perhaps previously took for granted'. In this sense, there was a clear distinction made between 'more able' and 'less able' older people. Thus, there was a strong association between disability and functional dependence (perceived as arising from bodily impairment rather than disabling barriers). In particular, older people were commonly viewed as disabled if they could not do certain things without assistance:

> Somebody who is just using a stick isn't necessarily in the same category as somebody who is in a wheelchair or housebound with the arthritis . . . They can function pretty well with a fairly small amount of assistance. So you cannot say every person who has got a mobility problem is in the same category of disability.

In functional terms, the visibility or nature of impairment became less important. For example, someone with heart disease was seen to be disabled, 'because they can't climb stairs, there's lot of things that they can't do. Just because its unseen, it's not visual, doesn't mean to say they're not disabled'. In this sense, 'Elderly people may be disabled whether or not they class themselves to be'. They were seen to be disabled because they 'become less able to maintain their own independence, reliant on other people, and become disabled'. This view was constructed, within some groups, with reference to their organisational ability to accommodate and support disabled people in their own service provision: for example, choosing only to cater to those older people who could 'look after themselves when they are here'.

The frequent use of physical or cognitive function as a determinant of both old age and disability led some groups of older people to be identified as ageing earlier than others, due to the early onset of age-related impairments associated with poverty, living and working conditions and so on (for example, those who were homeless). In particular, some organisations serving minority ethnic communities suggested that Black elders might experience illnesses associated with old age at a younger age than white people. Thus:

> The elders within the Black community actually suffer from illnesses, and ailments that are usually connected to people who are 60, 65 and over, which is our white counterparts ... So, rather than seeing age as just a number, we were actually targeting it to people who actually couldn't be as mobile as they were when they were younger, due to illnesses that are usually connected to old age.

The widespread construction of older people as those with functional impairments overlaid a more general theme in the data, connecting old age with loss of autonomy and with perceptions of dependence. Here, the key determinant was whether people could function autonomously or without assistance (i.e. 'independently'). This was also a key theme in the way that organisations talked about disability, providing the most obvious linkage between constructions of older people and disabled people. However, impairment was not the only reason why older people were seen to become less able to cope autonomously and bereavement (specifically the death of a spouse) was clearly identified as a trigger for change in similar terms.

There was then a widespread reliance on cultural associations between old age, disability and dependency. Becoming an older person was widely seen as a transition from a state of independence to one of dependence, frequently explained by reference to the onset of functional impairment. Here, the emphasis was not so much on the structural dependency of older people as a generational group but rather in terms of individual relationships of dependence upon others or upon services. This way of speaking belied an assumption that older people, and older disabled people in particular, were in some way deviating from a norm of autonomous physical functioning in everyday life that would otherwise have been available to them. In order to understand the significance of this position it is important to think carefully about the way in which we construct autonomy and independence. As I have argued elsewhere, the key to understanding this is to problematise our cultural and structural understanding of adulthood and autonomy (Priestley 2000).

A number of our interviewees emphasised the biographical disruption of impairment events in the process of becoming older (such as dementia, breaking a hip, angina, stroke, heart attack, life threatening illness, mental distress, depression, and so on). As one organisation put it, 'When people are fit and well, they don't feel elderly'. This construction of old age identity as precipitated by the onset of impairment accords with the frequent reference to impairment and chronic illness as 'biographical disruption' in medical sociology (Bury 1982), although Williams (2000) contests this view in relation to impairment acquired in old age (arguing that where the onset of impairment is accepted as part of a narrative of ageing the concept of disruption has less salience). Similarly, where Giddens (1991) highlights the 'ontological insecurity' of identity changes over the life course, Riggs and Turner (1997) suggest that the reality may be closer to a 'pragmatic accommodation' by individuals to everyday change over the life course.

As the preceding analysis suggests, we found little apparent awareness of the social model of disability among older people's groups (and there was no direct reference to this concept in any of the interviews or documentation). As one informant commented, 'I don't know how the disability movement would define it, I've never asked the question'. Rather, the construction of disability tended to reflect a more medico-functional model. Given the current high profile of social model rhetoric in policy making and advocacy with younger adults, this has significant implications for the disability movement, highlighting perhaps an apparent lack of disability equality and advocacy work with older people's organisations.

However, we did find some evidence of social model thinking in the definition of barriers facing older people with impairments. For example, 'someone who needs a hearing aid, without that aid, they would be disabled', or, 'We often ask if they can manage independently in the bathroom to bathe themselves and they'll often say well I could manage better if I had a bath seat or if I had a hand rail. So they might not necessarily be disabled because they are acquiring these things'. Consequently, there was some openness within organisations towards the view that disability might be contingent upon the removal of barriers and on available levels of support. Thus:

If it wasn't for our group they would be less able to do things that they wanted to do, to enjoy life or to have a quality of life, if they were to have to fend for themselves in this type of society. That sounds really quite awful really but the society that we live in is not very enabling.

Biography and identity

As mentioned previously, it was not our intention to talk directly to older people about their own identities with regard to disability and old age. However, our discussions revealed much that was relevant to these themes. There was, for example, a general consensus that older people tend to dissociate themselves from old age identity for as long as possible, and that the onset of impairment was a key factor in precipitating an individual's shift of willingness to identify as an older person (for example, by joining a group).

Biggs (1997) addresses the possibility of 'choosing not be old' within a context of postmodernity, drawing on Featherstone and Hepworth's (1991) concept of a 'mask of ageing' and psychodynamic concepts of masquerade. Featherstone, like Giddens (1991) argues that the uncertainties of high modernity threaten the maintenance of self-identity, particularly in the absence of clear guidelines for conveying people through the life course (requiring the continual and reflexive revision of biographical narrative during our lives). For Featherstone (or Bauman 1995) such uncertainties are perhaps better viewed as opportunities for reflexive identity choices drawing on an increasing array of cultural options. Moreover, and in contrast to the situation under modernity, such choices are viewed as largely separate, or at least distanced, from the material conditions of our lives, including the possibility to transcend or 'recode' the ageing body that 'masks' an inner more youthful self (Featherstone and Hepworth 1995). For Featherstone and Hepworth (1989) then, the 'mask' of ageing arises as the result of tensions between the ageing body and the ability to exercise consumer choices, bolstered by the attribution of negative qualities by others.

Biggs (1997) reviews these and other recent developments in identity theory in order to examine the identity management options for older people. Here, Biggs addresses the malleability of the ageing body with more scepticism, arguing that its limits and appearance do impose constraints and contradictions on attempts to present the supposed 'youthful self' within. However, Biggs also sees some possibilities for 'choosing not to be old', particularly in the rejection of stereotypes and the preservation of an adaptive self-identity:

> At root the problem would seem to centre on three themes; the nature of what is being hidden by masking, the role of the social environment in which masking takes place, and the importance of the body as a focus for conflict in identity management.   (Biggs 1997)

Thus, Biggs argues that the uncertainty of changing role expectations in old age offers possibilities as well as threats to the management of self (including the possibility of an ageless identity). However, it was clear from our research that key informants within organisations working with older people were much quicker to seize on the imperfect mask of the impaired body than on the identity within.

However, there were also counter-examples. In explaining why some people are more likely to resist identification with old age, our respondents often pointed to individual differences, life experience and motivation. As one informant put it: '. . . just because one person is 60 and another person 60, how they perceive themselves and how others perceive them is very different'. Personality factors and the desire to maintain a sense of 'independence' were common themes here, and most of our key informants argued that the people they targeted were likely to resist being labelled as older, for fear of being perceived as dependent (rather than leading active lives).

The desire to place distance between the idea of being older and the idea of being independent has been directly addressed in high profile 'active ageing' campaigns by national organisations representing older people (although there was no direct reference to this idea amongst the local groups we spoke to). Such campaigns have specifically sought to challenge the cultural association between older identities and perceived dependency, legitimising the inclusion of older people who might otherwise resist that labelling. Active ageing and the movement for the Third Age has been less about 'striving to be young', than about claiming positive old age identities (Featherstone and Hepworth 1995; Gibson 2000). Here, there are perhaps parallels with the kind of enabling disability identities claimed by many younger adults with impairments through the movement for independent living.

Disability, like old age, was sometimes viewed as an individual identity issue. As one group put it, people are disabled 'When they say they are disabled . . . the charity as a whole would encourage all of our staff not to make the decision for a person but to let the person make that decision themselves'. However, the emphasis was again on intrinsic personality factors and a motivation to remain independent:

> We have what I would consider to be really disabled older people who are active, involved, who push themselves despite their disabilities. We have others and the first sign of an ache or a pain that's enough to say, 'I won't be able to do this any more, or I need home care'.

Older disabled people, same or different?

Although disability was viewed variously, within medical, functional or social models, it was often seen to apply equally to people of all ages. Around half of the 21 organisations we visited considered everyone with significant impairment to be disabled, whether or not this was related to ageing – for example, '... whatever illness they have is disabling them from being able to take more social activities or quality of life they've had before', or, 'It's still a disability for an older person ... whether its old-age-related or not. It's still a disability in our eyes because they are disabled from doing something they want to do'. As another group told us: 'Just because people are getting older and physically less able does not mean they don't want to enjoy their lives ... As far as we are concerned, that is a disability'.

However, a similar proportion took a different view. For them, people with impairments acquired in old age, or normally associated with ageing, were not necessarily seen as disabled. For example:

> I would not necessarily say an older person had a disability if they have got age-related hearing loss. I would say well that's something that happens with age. It's like your hair going grey.

Similarly, one volunteer commented during an interview:

> I'm 66 and I have very bad arthritis ... also have high blood pressure, also have angina, also have under-active thyroid but there's no way I can consider myself disabled. I just consider that it's because I've got older.

The same logic was applied to functional as to medical definitions of disability. For example, people were not viewed as disabled where they were seen as able 'to carry out what *a normal elderly person* could do' (our emphasis). In this sense, the onset of certain forms of medical or functional impairment was not seen to deviate from preconceived norms of old age (i.e. as opposed to norms of adulthood). Nor were such impairments viewed as significant forms of biographical disruption to normative life course narratives of ageing. Rather, they were seen as an everyday part of the embodied generational habitus of old age (Turner 1989). To emphasise the point, there was a tendency to view disability in bodily and functional terms, and to construct disabled people as those outside the normal range *of their generational peers*.

Significantly, this seemed to suggest a widely held view of both impairment and disability as culturally situated within specific generational locations (i.e. that dynamic narratives of life course development and ageing can often override apparently static biomedical measurements of function and impairment in the construction of disability). In this sense, our respondents saw 'normal' levels of impairment in the ageing body as part of the habitus or the trappings of old age, and were resistant to the idea of thinking about older people with such impairments as disabled. In many ways this was quite a positive thing and encouraged the inclusion of many people with impairments in mainstream activities and services for older people. On the negative side, it meant that such organisations had often failed to consider the barriers faced by older disabled people in terms of disability rights that would almost certainly have been apparent in services to younger people with similar impairments.

Note

This chapter draws on research arising from a small project grant and a three-year research fellowship, both funded by the UK Economic and Social Research Council (award numbers R000223581 and R000271078).

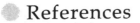 # References

Bauman, Z. (1995) *Life in Fragments: essays in postmodern morality*, Blackwell, Oxford.

Biggs, S. (1997) 'Choosing not to be old? Masks, bodies and identity management in later life', *Ageing and Society*, **17**, pp. 553–570.

Blaikie, A. (1999) *Ageing and Popular Culture*, Cambridge University Press, Cambridge.

Bury, M. (1982) 'Chronic Illness as Biographical Disruption', *Sociology of Health and Illness*, **4**(2), pp. 167–182.

Corker, M. (2001) *Disabling Language: analyzing disability discourse*, Routledge, London.

Corker, M. and French, S.E. (1999) *Disability Discourse*, Open University Press, Milton Keynes.

Dutton, K. (1996) *The Perfectible Body*, Cassell, London.

Featherstone, M. and Hepworth, M. (1989) 'Ageing and old age; reflections on the postmodern lifecourse' in Bytheway, B., Kiel, T., Allat, P. and Bryman, A. (eds) *Becoming and Being Old*, Sage, London.

Featherstone, M. and Hepworth, M. (1991) 'The mask of ageing and the postmodern lifecourse' in Featherstone, M., Hepworth, M. and Turners, B. (eds) *The Body, Social Process and Cultural Theory*, Sage, London.

Featherstone, M. and Hepworth, M. (1995) 'Images of positive ageing' in Featherstone, M. and Wernick, A. (eds) *Images of Ageing*, Routledge, London.

Finkelstein, V. (1991) 'Disability: an Administrative Challenge? (the health and welfare heritage)' in Oliver, M. (ed.) *Social Work: disabled people and disabling environments*, Jessica Kingsley, London.

Gibson, H.B. (2000) 'It keeps us young', *Ageing and Society*, **20**, pp. 773–779.

Giddens, A. (1991) *Modernity and Self Identity: Self and Society in the Late Modern Age*, Polity Press, Cambridge.

Gilleard, C. and Higgs, P. (1998) 'Ageing and the limiting conditions of the body', *Sociological Research Online*, **3**(4), pp. U56–U70.

Hughes, B. and Paterson, K. (1997) 'The Social Model of Disability and the Disappearing Body: towards a sociology of impairment', *Disability and Society*, **12**(3), pp. 325–340.

Katz, S. (1996) *Disciplining Old Age: the formation of gerontological knowledge*, University of Virginia Press, Charlottesville, VA.

Laslett, P. (1989) *A Fresh Map of Life: the emergence of the third age*, Weidenfeld and Nicolson, London.

Minkler, M. and Estes, C. (eds) (1991) *Critical Perspectives on Aging: the political and moral economy of growing old*, Baywood Press, Amityville, NY.

Oberg, P. (1996) 'The absent body – a social gerontological paradox', *Ageing and Society*, **16**, pp. 701–719.

Oliver, M. (1990) *The Politics of Disablement*, Macmillan, Basingstoke.

Phillipson, C. (1982) *Capitalism and the construction of old age*, Macmillan, London.

Priestley, M. (2000) 'Adults only: Disability, social policy and the life course', *Journal of Social Policy*, **29**, pp. 421–439.

Priestley, M. (ed.) (2001) *Disability and the Life Course: global perspectives*, Cambridge University Press, Cambridge.

Priestley, M. (2002) 'Whose Voices? Representing the claims of older disabled people under New Labour', *Policy and Politics*, **30**(3), pp. 361–373.

Priestley, M. and Rabiee, P. (2001) *Building Bridges: disability and old age*, University of Leeds, final report of ESRC research project R000223581, Leeds.

Riggs, A. and Turner, B.S. (1997) 'The sociology of the postmodern self: Intimacy, identity and emotions in adult life', *Australian Journal on Ageing*, **16**(4), pp. 229–232.

Thompson, P., Itzin, C. and Abendstern, M. (1990) *I Don't Feel Old: the experience of later life*, Oxford University Press, Oxford.

Turner, B. (1989) 'Ageing, Politics and Sociological Theory', *British Journal of Sociology*, **40**(4), pp. 588–606.

Williams, S. (2000) 'Chronic illness as biographical disruption or biographical disruption as chronic illness? Reflections on a core concept' in *Sociology of Health and Illness*, **22**(1), pp. 40–67.

Ylanne-McEwen, V. (1999) '"Young at heart": discourses of age identity in travel agency interaction', *Ageing and Society*, **19**, pp. 417–440.

CHAPTER 5

Challenging a 'spoiled identity': mental health service users, recognition and redistribution

Iain Ferguson

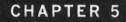 ## Introduction

For close to two decades, notions of identity and difference have provided the primary bases of organisation and mobilisation for those wishing to challenge injustices and inequalities within Western capitalist societies (Woodward 1997). The growth of identity-based movements during this period can be seen as a product of the widespread disillusionment of the 'Children of '68' with the class-based movements to challenge successfully the citadels of capital during the 1960s and 1970s (Harman 1988). The emergence of new movements during the 1980s and 1990s around issues such as sexuality or disability can also be seen more positively, however, as products of what has been called 'the radicalised Enlightenment':

> Ideals that were intended initially to have quite a narrow reference, to benefit primarily white men of property, proved capable of indefinite extension. The result is a process of permanent revolution, in which a procession of new political subjects – workers, slaves, women, colonial subjects, people of colour, oppressed nationalities, lesbians and gays, disabled people . . . – emerge to stake their claim to the liberty and equality won by earlier struggles.   (Callinicos 2000, p. 24)

This chapter will seek to assess the usefulness of notions of identity and difference in understanding the experience of one of these new movements – the mental health service users' movement (Rogers and Pilgrim 1991). The chapter is largely based on individual interviews and group discussions with a total of eighty mental health service users and twenty workers in fourteen community-based mental health projects across Central Scotland during 1997 and 1998 (Ferguson 1999, from now on referred to as 'the Scottish research'). The majority of those interviewed were involved in the management and development of the organisations to which they belonged, usually as secretaries, chairpersons or committee members, in some cases at a national level. In that sense, they formed part of the 'cadre' of the mental health users' movement in Scotland. All had extensive experience of the mental health system, with more than 75 per cent having been hospitalised at some point and just under half having been given a diagnosis of schizophrenia or manic depression. The aim of the interviews was to explore the identities of mental health service users.

The main part of the chapter will focus on cultural/ideological issues within the mental health service users' movement, through an exploration of debates within the movement over terminology. On the basis of that discussion, the usefulness of notions of diverse identities as a basis for understanding the users' movement will be critically assessed, drawing in part on Nancy Fraser's critique of identity politics, including its alleged propensities for *reification* of identities and *displacement* of issues of redistribution (Fraser 1995, p. 2000). Finally, in contrast to the 'freefloating', self-defining nature of much current identity theorising, it will be suggested that it is necessary to ground both the misrecognition, or stigma, that users experience, and also the material injustices which they suffer, within the specific economic and social relations of capitalism.

Challenging a 'spoiled identity'

In an earlier study, Rogers and Pilgrim noted that *experience*, both of the mental health system and of mental ill-health *per se*, was the most common reason given by respondents for becoming involved in selfhelp or campaigning activities (Rogers and Pilgrim 1991). In this section, through a discussion of language and terminology, I wish to look at the way in which users had *constructed* this experience and the extent to which these constructions challenged or undermined dominant ideologies of mental ill-health, whether biomedical or populist. Challenges to a 'spoiled identity' (Goffman 1963) which seek to replace it with a more

Table 5.1 Preferred terminology for people with mental health problems

preferred term	user respondents
'patient'	4
'user'	7
'customer'	2
'client'	2
'survivor'	8
'member'	3
'more than one'	4
'other'	12

positive identity might be seen as a first step by service users in challenging the wider stigma and oppression they experience. Historically, such challenges have often been reflected in the language of the 'movements' – in the shift from 'Negro' to 'black' in the US civil rights movement in the 1960s, for example, or from 'homosexual' to 'gay' in the later gay rights movement. An examination of changing terminology amongst users of mental health services may therefore provide a useful indicator to some of the issues of identity referred to above.

Table 5.1 shows the responses of forty-two service users in the Scottish study when asked in individual interviews to select their preferred term from the following terms printed on a card: *patient, client, survivor, customer, user, other.*

In this section, each of these answers will be briefly discussed and followed by a more general discussion of their significance.

Patient

Psychiatry is more than just a branch of medicine. It is a vast edifice with an ideology, an attitude, and most of all, it is a language which shapes the reality it claims to describe.   (Kotowicz 1997, p. 12)

While Kotowicz overstates the case (the 'reality' of psychiatric practice is at least as powerfully shaped by other, more material factors, such as the role of the drug companies), nevertheless it is true that the social construction of disturbances in thought, feeling and behaviour as forms and symptoms of *illness*, and its accompanying language – the biomedical model of mental illness – has enjoyed virtually total hegemony in the area of mental distress for more than one hundred and fifty years (Busfield 1986).

Despite that dominance, however, only four out of 42 respondents in this study selected 'patient', the term most closely associated with this model, as their preferred term. Of those who did, for at least one respondent, this clearly reflected not a positive choice but rather an ambivalent recognition of what she perceived to be the realities of the situation:

> The overall focus is still on symptoms and illness and treatment. As someone with a mental illness, I tend to feel I've been labelled a patient forever. I'm so against labelling – I'm just someone with an illness.
>
> (Survivors' Poetry Scotland)

For others, 'patient' was seen as an appropriate term within the hospital setting, but inappropriate in other contexts. For a worker with one project: 'The term patient would only apply in the context of treatment.'

For a member of Survivors' Poetry, the term was 'too passive' while a Stepping Stones respondent felt it was 'too dependency-oriented'. One MDFS member felt it had connotations that 'you'll wait while someone else does something', while for another MDFS respondent, '"patient" suggests the person can't help themselves'.

For others, the term connoted what Foucault has described as 'the clinical gaze . . . a surveillance that makes it possible to qualify, to classify and to punish. It establishes over individuals a visibility through which one differentiates and judges them' (cited in Parton 1991, pp. 6–7):

> Patient is much more medical – it plays into the idea of seeing someone in the context of their illness, rather than as a person in their own right.
>
> (Survivors' Poetry Scotland)

Amongst those rejecting the term, however, the most common reason given was the power imbalance it implied:

> Client and patient both head towards a disempowered status.
>
> (Scottish Users' Network)
>
> Patient? No, that's a power thing.   (Core Club)

Customer

Consumerist discourses – the service user as customer – have been extremely influential within policy discussions of service user involvement over the past decade (Clarke 1998). It can with justification be described as the 'official model' of service user involvement, since its prescriptions have been enshrined in the NHS and Community Care Act and in subsequent policy guidance. One might assume then that many users would have been persuaded to see themselves as customers. In fact, in the Scottish study, only two interviewees responded positively to the term:

> I quite like 'customer', I like the implications. Personally, I feel that all services should be person-centred. The person in hospital or wherever is the person with the income on his head and should be seen as such.
>
> (GANET)

For other respondents, however, the term was variously seen as too commercially-orientated, politically conservative or simply inappropriate:

> 'Customer' is not appropriate – we don't have choices. (SUN)
>
> 'Customer' is not a word I'd use very often – usually in relation to BT. (GANET)
>
> 'Customer' is meaningless. If we were given sufficient money, then we might be customers. (SUN)

It seems that the realities of users' day-to-day experience of lack of resources and lack of choice may outweigh attempts by government to reconstruct them as consumers of mental health services.

User

The term 'user' or 'service user' is now commonly used to refer to people who are receiving services from health and social services. How did the respondents in the Scottish study view the term? An Executive member of SUN concisely summed up what he saw as the strengths and limitations of the term as follows:

> On a more general level, we use users because it's more commonly used. It has two advantages. Firstly, it's less exclusive. Survivor implies having survived both the mental health system and also survived mental health problems. People are at different stages and some don't yet feel that they have survived their mental health problems. Emotionally, I prefer survivor but user is less exclusive – like trade unionist, it's more role-specific. Its disadvantage is that there are many services that people don't *use* at all but are *abused* by them – that's a contradiction in reality. 'User' implies you can be an actor *and* a user of services. In that sense it can be seen as positive i.e. what we would like to be.   (SUN)

Another group of respondents saw the term in a very different light however. In contrast to the SUN respondent above, 'user' implied passivity:

> I don't like the word 'user' because as users we're not putting anything in.   (Core Club)
>
> 'User' has connotations and does not allow people to escape services... I don't like the passivity of 'user' or the others.
>   (Worker, Stepping Stones.)

For others, it was these connotations that made the word unacceptable:

> The general public doesn't understand 'user' – it's associated with drug abuse.   (Survivors' Poetry Scotland)

Survivor

For some of those respondents who disliked the term 'user', 'survivor' offered a more positive alternative.

> The term I use to describe my own experience is 'survivor' – and that's about surviving the mental health system. In my work, I use 'user' – the majority of people will use services at some point.   (SUN)

> I like 'survivor'. My favourite saying is 'We're still here – we've survived.' A lot of the people who have been through this project have had horrendous pasts. But we're here, we've got here – we wouldn't be here if we hadn't.   (Stepping Stones)

The ambiguities of the term were concisely summed up by the following respondent:

> If I had to plump for one term, it would be 'survivor'... 'survivor' has a good ring to it. In Survivors' Poetry, the word means more than just a user of mental health services. It includes anyone who has had any kind of trauma in their lives, such as abuse, and also people with disabilities. 'Patient' and 'client' are too passive. 'Customer' is too commercial. However, in the Survivors' Poetry Scotland letterhead, it talks about 'survivors of the mental health system'. I think that might be counter-productive. There is a possibility that some people might think it means that the whole mental health system is wrong and destructive. I don't feel that. I am a survivor of mental illness and have had positive experiences of the mental health system as well as damaging experiences. It's a strong ongoing debate.
> (Survivors' Poetry Scotland)

As with 'user', however, there were those for whom the term had negative connotations:

> 'Survivor' I hate. You've survived as in you're still living but not as you should be. It implies you've come out the other end – I haven't.
> (Stepping Stones)

> I don't like 'survivor' – I see it as a slightly aggressive term, that there is a system that people have come through. That's against them. It's rather aggressive.   (GANET)

Client

The term 'client' was rarely a first choice and where it was suggested, it was normally qualified by a 'maybe' or a 'probably'. Where it was seen positively, this was because it was seen either as a fairly neutral term or alternatively as appropriate in the specific context of counselling activities. For others, however, the connotations of 'client' with social work services made it a less acceptable term:

> Patient and client are too passive.   (Survivors' Poetry Scotland)
>
> Client has become quite a negative term – the social work equivalent to policing – and is discredited.   (SUN)

As Table 5.1 indicated, almost a third of respondents either opted for a term not on the card provided or found none of the terms satisfactory. These alternative suggestions are interesting in highlighting the wide range of ideas currently being debated within the users' movement.

Member

Interestingly, in the context of a discussion of identity issues, the only term to which no respondent objected was 'member'. All of the projects in the study referred to their 'members'. Whereas the other terms may be seen as conferring an identity, as defining an individual in terms of their mental health experience, membership confers no such permanent identity; it is less *essentialist* than the other terms (Woodward 1997). One chooses to join a club or organisation and one may choose to leave; one may choose also to join a host of other organisations at the same time. 'Member' is also the term employed within the growing International Clubhouse Association to which the Core Club is affiliated and a worker there explained the rationale for using the term:

> Here, it's 'members'. I'm not keen on the term 'user'. Other than in the club, just 'people'. 'Member' has to do with ownership and there's also no stigma. I find the term quite empowering and it doesn't say you're using 'the services' or are going to be using them all your life. Ex-patients who instigated the Core Club decided on the term.

Person with the diagnosis

The term 'person with the diagnosis' was suggested by members of one organisation – Manic Depression Fellowship Scotland – and was unusual in that most respondents in this study were hostile to an emphasis on diagnosis which they saw as being the basis of labelling on the one hand and as obscuring the shifting nature of mental ill-health as a process on the other. For some MDFS members, however, to speak of 'someone with the diagnosis' was seen as having the advantage of separating the person from the condition in a way which the other terms did not do:

> Someone who doesn't accept the medical diagnosis is in denial. It's the person who has the diagnosis. Someone with epilepsy, for example, is a person with epilepsy, not an epileptic. (MDFS)

Madperson

At the other end of the linguistic spectrum, the term 'madperson' was mentioned positively by some SUN respondents:

> There are other terms like 'mad' – equivalent to the use of 'dykes' in the gay and lesbian movement. That's the most enjoyable term – especially with psychiatrists. I think it's great to use the word 'mad' – we have 'Glad to be Mad' tee-shirts. 'Mad' also has the double meaning of 'angry'. 'Mad' has lost much of its former stigma – 'mentally ill' and 'insane' now carry that stigma. (SUN member)

The belief that terms of oppression can be 'appropriated' by the oppressed and turned against the oppressor is a fairly common one within a number of the 'new social movements'. The leading organisation of gay men in the USA, after all, is Queer Nation, the name a conscious 'appropriation' of a term of anti-homosexual abuse. At one level, it can be argued that such an attempt to appropriate the language of oppression represents a defiant and admirable refusal to accept the stigma implicit in certain terms. A high point of the popular 1996 television series 'Taking Over the Asylum', for example, was a demonstration organised by psychiatric patients under the slogan 'We are loonies and we are proud'. Against this, it has been argued that not only does using such 'politically correct' language often reflect an exaggerated belief in the power of language to change people's actual living conditions but it may also be regarded by most people as an *acceptance* of oppression, rather than a means of challenging it (Smith 1994). In respect of mental health service users, there is the additional issue of the extent to which it is possible to embrace a 'user' identity in the same way as a gay or black identity, an issue to which we shall return later.

No suitable term

Finally, there were those who saw no term as being particularly useful. As Table 5.1 indicates, this constituted the largest group of respondents but even those individuals who did opt for a particular term often did so reluctantly. The following comments are fairly typical:

> 'People with mental health difficulties' is in some ways the best of all – it covers a wide range of people.   (SUN)
>
> This is one of the debates I'm engaged in. There's no clear answer. If I had to plump for one term, it would be 'survivor'. None of these terms is satisfactory.   (Survivors' Poetry Scotland)

Implicit in the above comments was the recognition that each of these terms might simply be a new 'label' which continued to define people primarily in terms of their mental health problems.

Towards a mental health identity?

What conclusions can be drawn from the above discussion of changing terminology? At the most general level, the discussion appears to highlight the *transitional* nature of both mental health services and mental health ideologies. As Barham and Hayward have noted, the era of the 'career mental patient' may be over but as yet it is not clear what will replace it (Barham and Hayward 1995).

Changing ideas amongst mental health service users, in other words, reflect at least in part the shift in mental health provision from the asylum to 'the community', however defined. The influence of ideas from other social movements, such as the gay movement or the disability movement, is also evident.

In terms of the *content* of the ideas discussed above, two points in particular seem to stand out. On the one hand, there is the rejection by these respondents of the disempowering aspects of the biomedical model of mental ill-health, as reflected, for example, in the criticisms of the term 'patient'. It might have been assumed that with the decline of the asylum, this model would in any event become less influential but this may prove to be a questionable assumption. Certainly within the US context, far from loosening the grip of biomedical psychiatry, the process of 'deinstitutionalisation' has strengthened it reflecting in part the influence of multinational drug companies (Breggin 1993). In Britain, the 'hospital in the community' model of mental health community care also appears to be gaining ground (Rogers *et al.* 1993). At the same time, it should be noted that what is primarily being rejected by the respondents in this study is the *dominance* of this model and the *power relations* it entails, rather than biomedical involvement or expertise *per se*. Many users saw a continuing role for mental health professionals and treatments but within a more holistic, partnership-based mental health service.

The second notable point arising from the discussion is the lack of consensus regarding a preferred term for people with mental health problems. As well as reflecting the current transitional state of mental health services and of mental health ideologies referred to above, it may also be that the lack of an agreed term reflects more profound issues about the nature of 'a mental health identity'. This may have implications for the applicability of identity politics in general and a social model of health in particular to mental health users. Some of these issues are briefly discussed below.

A positive identity?

A common practice of recent social movements has been to invert a previously stigmatised or devalued characteristic, relating to skin colour or gender or sexual orientation for example, and claim it as the basis for a new and positive identity. Obvious examples would include slogans such as 'Black Power' or 'Gay Pride'. It is less easy, however, to 'reclaim' mental ill-health, however conceptualised, in this way. As Sedgwick noted, for virtually all psychiatric schools, whether Freudian, Jungian or biomedical, mental ill-health in general, and psychosis in particular, is 'breakdown, sheer affliction' (Sedgwick 1982, p. 98), while even R.D. Laing in his later writings argued:

I never idealized mental suffering, or romanticised despair, dissolution, torture or terror ... I have never denied the existence of patterns of mind and conduct that are excruciating.   (Laing 1985, pp. 8–9)

Even the language of mental ill-health or mental distress is evaluative, as neither mental illness nor mental distress (the term more commonly used within the users' movement) are usually regarded as desirable or sought-after states. Within this study, there was an implicit assumption (as well as many explicit statements) on the part of most, if not all, respondents that mental ill-health *impaired* functioning at the level of feeling, cognition, and behaviour. Hence the limits of 'Glad to be Mad'. Mental ill-health for these respondents was a state which might be learned from but hardly one to be actively sought.

A permanent identity?

Members of other social movements have tended to base identity on an *enduring* characteristic such as skin colour or gender or disability. By contrast, for the majority of people who experience mental ill-health, it is likely to be of a *transient* nature. Even for those in this study who experienced frequent relapses, mental ill-health was nevertheless a process from 'good health' to 'ill-health' and back again. Hence the dissatisfaction expressed by some respondents regarding the term 'survivor'. It implied a finality or resolution that they did not recognise. On the positive side, it was the fluctuating nature of mental ill-health that allowed many users (or former users) to play a major role in running organisations, and also provided the basis for a critique of medical labelling which saw people as always ill. From the perspective of identity politics, however, this lack of permanence plus the very real stigma associated with mental ill-health, means that few are likely to wish to 'come out' as service users, let alone be identified as permanent 'users', committed to the building of a users' movement. To do so would be to risk job, house, family and friendships.

Social construct or immanent condition?

Woodward has suggested a polarisation in current social theory between those who see identities as socially constructed and those who see them as rooted in biology (Woodward 1997). The current discussion would suggest that, as far as making sense of mental ill-health goes, neither of these polarities is adequate. As Barham and Hayward argue in their discussion of the issues facing mental health users in the community, 'neither biological reductionism nor an exclusive social constructivism constitute viable intellectual positions' (Barham and Hayward 1995, p. 167). As the discussion around the term 'survivor' indicates, for example, being a 'person with a mental health problem' involves *both* social construct *and* individual experience with profound implications for social functioning, some of which are socially constructed, others of which flow from the experience itself. The issue for the respondents in this study was not *whether* help was needed when people were experiencing mental distress but rather the *type* of help that was on offer and the power relations within which it was offered. As the discussion around the term 'patient' suggests, the clash identified by service users is often between the personal experience of distress and the professional construction of that distress, a distinction which Barham and Hayward correctly describe as enormously important (Barham and Hayward 1995).

A shared identity?

For Woodward, identity politics:

involves claiming one's identity as a member of [a] marginalised group as a political point of departure and thus identity becomes a major factor in political mobilization.   (Woodward 1997, p. 24)

In essence, this approach involves singling out one aspect of one's experience, such as gender or sexual orientation, and making that the basis of a shared identity. In respect of mental ill-health, the above discussion highlights the difficulties in agreeing on what constitutes a 'shared identity' for people with mental health problems. Who, in other words, is a 'user'? On the one hand, one could adopt a *broadly*-based definition of a mental health identity, based purely on the *experience* of mental ill-health and/or using 'services', however defined; on the other, 'user' could be defined far more exclusively, on the basis of having been hospitalised, for example, or of having a psychotic condition. If one adopts the first definition, one would include between a seventh and a quarter of the population of Britain; if the latter, one risks excluding millions of people who are by any criterion experiencing mental distress, while at the same time basing the movement on the•most disabled people.

Rethinking identity?

Two major issues emerge from the discussion so far. On the one hand, there is clearly profound dissatisfaction on the part of these service users with the ways in which their experience is currently appropriated and classified by others, particularly by psychiatric professionals. At the same time, the points raised in the previous section suggest that notions of identity and difference may have limited value as a basis for challenging the stigma and oppression which people with mental health problems experience. While some of the limitations of such theorising arise from the specific characteristics of this particular group of people – the transient nature of mental ill-health, for example – recent discussions of identity and difference suggest that the difficulties with these notions as a basis for challenging oppression and stigma are more deep-rooted.

The political theorist Nancy Fraser has distinguished between what she sees as two analytically distinct forms of justice, one of which is concerned with *redistribution*, the other with *recognition* (Fraser 1995, 2000). The first is socio-economic injustice, which is rooted in the political-economic structure of capitalism and gives rise to struggles for redistribution. Examples of this form of injustice include exploitation, economic marginalisation and deprivation. The second kind of justice is cultural or symbolic and, Fraser argues, includes

cultural domination (being subjected to patterns of interpretation and communication that are associated with another culture and are alien and/or hostile to one's own); nonrecognition (being rendered invisible via the authoritative representational, communicative and interpretative practices of one's own culture); and disrespect (being routinely maligned or disparaged in stereotypic public cultural representations and/or in everyday life interactions).   (Fraser 1995, p. 71)

This form of injustice gives rise to 'struggles for recognition', which in recent years have typically taken the form of struggles over difference, based on what Fraser calls 'the identity model' (Fraser 2000, p. 109).

'Struggles for redistribution' will be discussed below, but the relevance of Fraser's second form of injustice – the denial of recognition – to users of mental health services is obvious. Charles Taylor's comments on this form of injustice could well have been written with mental health service users in mind:

> Nonrecognition or misrecognition . . . can be a form of oppression, imprisoning someone in a false, distorted reduced mode of being. Beyond simple lack of respect, it can inflict a grievous wound, saddling people with crippling self-hatred. Due recognition is not just a courtesy but a vital human need.
>
> (Taylor, cited in Fraser 1995, p. 71)

The 'nonrecognition' or 'misrecognition' of people with mental health problems, whether by well-intentioned mental health professionals who reduce the lived experience of their patients to a set of biochemical processes, or by a tabloid press intent on emphasising their alleged 'dangerousness' is well-documented and often extreme (Philo 1996; SAMH 1999; Sayce 2000). Not surprisingly, such negative stereotypes are often internalised by people with mental health problems themselves. Warner cites studies showing that mental patients are as negative in their opinions of mental illness as is the general public and in some cases were even *more* rejecting of people with mental health problems than were family members or hospital staff (Warner 1994, p. 181). Given the prevalence of such a 'spoiled identity', the 'struggle for recognition' has a particularly profound meaning for this group of people which goes beyond demands for citizenship: it is the struggle to be recognised as fully human.

Fraser's concern is not to deny the impact of such misrecognition on people's health and self-esteem nor the importance of what she calls 'struggles for recognition' but is rather to expose the limitations of identity politics as a basis for both understanding and challenging such misrecognition For Fraser, what she labels the 'identity model' suffers from two main weaknesses: *reification of identity* and *displacement of redistribution*. Each of these will be considered below in terms of their relevance for mental health service users.

i Reification of identity

Identity politics, Fraser argues, through its stress on the need for those who share a particular characteristic or experience to display 'an authentic, self-affirming and self-generated collective identity' tends to promote conformism, to discourage disagreement or debate and to mask divisions within the group. As she argues:

> The overall effect is to impose a single, drastically simplified group-identity which denies the complexity of people's lives, the multiplicity of their identifications and the crosspull of their various affiliations.
>
> (Fraser 2000, p. 112)

We have seen above the difficulty of trying to reduce the experience of mental health service users to a single 'mental health identity'. In addition, Fraser argues, an emphasis on a shared identity can discourage attempts to explore other intragroup divisions such as gender, sexuality and class. Conversely, although not mentioned by Fraser, an emphasis on a single characteristic or experience as a basis for a shared identity can lead oppressed groups to embrace bedfellows whose material interests are often very different from their own (as in the attempt, for example, by some groups of mental health service users to claim Sir Winston Churchill, life-long eugenicist and ruling-class militant, as a fellow survivor (Ferguson 2000)). For Fraser, however, the main division which is ignored as a result of this 'reification of identity' is class division and it is this neglect which forms the basis of her second criticism of identity politics.

ii Displacement of redistribution

> Largely silent on the subject of economic inequality, the identity model treats misrecognition as a free-standing cultural harm: many of its proponents simply ignore distributive injustices altogether and focus exclusively on efforts to change culture; others, in contrast, appreciate the seriousness of maldistribution and genuinely wish to redress it. Yet both currents end by displacing redistributive claims.
>
> (Fraser 2000, p. 110)

Fraser is making a number of important points here which require some comment. First, she notes the silence of adherents and theorists of identity politics on the issue of class inequality. The failure of the identity model to account for such material inequality clearly raises serious questions about its usefulness both as explanatory paradigm and also as theoretical foundation for challenging oppression. As I have argued elsewhere, class inequality shapes every aspect of the lives of mental health service users (Ferguson 2000): in Brandon's phrase, 'poverty is the most common symptom of mental illness' (Brandon 1991, p. 32)

Second, there is the tendency within identity politics to view issues of misrecognition as 'free-floating'. Fraser again:

> The roots of injustice are located in demeaning representations but these are not seen as socially grounded. For this current, the nub of the problem is free-floating discourses, not *institutionalized* signification and norms. Hypostasizing culture, they both abstract misrecognition from its institutional matrix and obscure its entwinement with distributive injustice ... Obfuscating such connexions, they strip misrecognition of its social-structural underpinnings and equate it with distorted identity.
> (Fraser 2000, pp. 110–111)

If there is no link between discourses and material circumstances, it is difficult to explain why ideas about mental ill-health should have *changed* over the past two decades both amongst service users (as the above discussion suggests they have) and also the wider public (SAMH 1999). Similarly, it is difficult to explain the growth of notions of 'dangerousness' in relation to mental health during the 1990s without reference to the scapegoating tendencies of both Conservative and New Labour governments during the 1990s (Ferguson 1994; Lavalette and Mooney 2000).

Moreover, a focus primarily on cultural issues is likely to lead to a neglect of the *material* issues, such as jobs and houses, which numerous studies, including the largest study of service users' views (Rogers, Pilgrim and Lacey 1993) have shown that users see as central.

Fraser's third criticism is directed against those adherents of the identity model who *do* see issues of redistribution as important but who, seeing the cultural as material, believe that by changing ideas and cultural practices, this will lead to a change in the distribution of resources. As she rightly comments:

> In this way, culturalist proponents of identity politics simply reverse the claims of an earlier form of vulgar Marxist economism: they allow the politics of recognition to displace the politics of redistribution, just as vulgar Marxism once allowed the politics of redistribution to displace the politics of recognition. In fact, vulgar culturalism is no more adequate for understanding society than vulgar economism was.
>
> (Fraser 2000, p. 111)

While space does not permit a discussion of Fraser's own (Weberian) solution to the relationship between recognition and redistribution, what the above quotation suggests is that simply challenging stigmatising ideas is not enough and that what is necessary is to challenge *both* stigmatising ideas and cultural practices *and* the social and economic relationships that underpin these ideas and practices.

Conclusion: the limits of difference

I began this chapter by suggesting that notions of identity and difference had been central both to social theory and to popular struggles for the best part of two decades. The chapter's focus on changing terminology within the mental health users' movement has meant, however, that the discussion has been primarily around *identity* and its relevance (or lack of relevance) to the struggles of mental health service users. In closing, however, it is necessary to say a word or two about *difference*. Specifically, I want to suggest that an emphasis on difference may be even less helpful for mental health service users than an emphasis on a shared identity, for three main reasons.

First, as we saw in the discussion above on the limitations of a mental health identity, the difficulties faced by other oppressed groups in seeking to challenge discrimination and oppression are, if anything, even greater for mental health service users, as a consequence both of the depth of stigma that they experience and also of their recurrent mental ill-health. Their need for powerful allies is consequently at least as great as that of other oppressed groups. An emphasis on difference (as opposed to a recognition of diversity) may not be the best basis for building such alliances.

Second, an emphasis on the uniqueness of the experience of mental health service users fails to do justice to the ubiquity of mental ill-health in contemporary capitalist society. For example, an International Labour Organisation report into workplace-related mental health problems in several European countries noted that in the USA, clinical depression affects one in ten working age adults each year resulting in a loss of approximately 200 million working days, while in Britain, each year nearly three out of every ten employees experience mental health problems (ILO 2000). Similarly, stress was identified by 6,000 health and safety representatives in a TUC survey as the single major health and safety issue experienced by workers (TUC 1998).

It may suit the interests of the tabloid press and of unprincipled politicians to portray people with mental health problems as 'different' from the rest of 'us', but what these figures suggest is that the users' movement is on much stronger ground in emphasising the *commonness* of mental ill-health.

Finally, these figures point to another important fact: that the distribution and extent of mental health problems is not chance or random but reflects the wider distribution of power and resources within our society. Brown and Harris, in a classic study of the relationship between mental ill-health and social inequality, reported that working-class women are four times more likely to experience clinical depression than their middle-class counterparts. These findings, they suggest:

> ...have implications that concern not only the optimum organisation of the family but also the role of women in the wider economy and the values given these functions by the media and society at large.
> (Brown and Harris 1978, p. 291)

What this indicates is that there is – potentially, at least – much scope for common cause between the struggles of mental health service users against stigma, oppression and social inequality and the struggles of other oppressed groups and trade unionists against their particular oppressions and exploitation. It would be wrong to suggest that building such alliances will be an easy task, especially given the depth of stigma which currently exists towards people with mental health problems. The successes of both the gay movement and the disability movement over the past decade in challenging stigma and creating powerful alliances suggests, however, that that task, though difficult, is far from being impossible.

Appendix – Organisations involved in the Scottish Research

Individual Interviews:
- Survivors' Poetry Scotland
- The Core Club, Dumfermline
- Stepping Stones, Clydebank.
- Saheliya, Edinburgh.
- Charlie Reid Centre, Glasgow.
- AdvoCard, Edinburgh.
- Glasgow Advocacy Network (GANET)
- Scottish Users' Network (SUN)
- Manic Depression Fellowship Scotland (MDFS)

Focus Groups:
- Ayr Action
- Edinburgh Users' Forum
- Fife Mental Health Survivors Group
- Eastwood Users' Forum
- People Need People (Falkirk)

References

Barham, P. and Hayward, R. (1995) *Relocating Madness: From the Mental Patient to the Person*, Free Association, London.

Barnes, C. and Mercer, G. (eds) (1996) *Exploring the Divide: Illness and Disability*, The Disability Press, Leeds.

Bradley, H. (2000) 'Social inequalities: coming to term with complexity' in Browning, G., Halcli, A. and Webster, F. (eds) *Understanding Contemporary Society: Theories of the Present*, Sage, London.

Brandon, D. (1991) *Innovation without Change? Consumer power in the psychiatric services*, Macmillan, Basingstoke.

Breggin, P. (1993) *Toxic Psychiatry*, HarperCollins, London.

Brown, G. and Harris, T. (1978) *Social Origins of Depression: a study of psychiatric disorder in women*, Tavistock, London.

Busfield, J. (1986) *Managing Madness – Changing Ideas and Practice*, Hutchinson, London.

Callinicos, A. (2000) *Equality*, Polity, London.

Clarke, J. (1998) 'Consumerism' in Hughes, G. (ed.) *Imagining Welfare Futures*, Routledge/Open University, London.

Ferguson, I. (1994) 'Containing the Crisis: crime and the Tories', *International Socialism*, **62**, pp. 51–70.

Ferguson, I. (1999) *The Potential and Limits of Mental Health Service User Involvement*, unpublished Ph.D. thesis, University of Glasgow.

Ferguson, I. (2000) 'Identity Politics or Class Struggle? The case of the mental health users' movement' in Lavalette, M. and Mooney, G. (eds) *Class Struggle and Welfare*, Routledge, London.

Fraser, N. (1995) 'From Redistribution to Recognition? Dilemmas of Justice in a "Post-Socialist" Age', *New Left Review*, 212, pp. 68–92.

Fraser, N. (2000) 'Rethinking Recognition', *New Left Review*, 3, pp. 107–120.

Goffman, E. (1963) *Stigma: Notes on the management of Spoiled Identity*, Penguin, Harmondsworth.

Halcli, A. and Webster, F. (eds) *Understanding Contemporary Society: Theories of the Present*, Sage, London.

Harman, C. (1988) *The Fire Last Time: 1968 and After*, Bookmarks, London.

ILO (2000) *Mental Health in the Workplace*, ILO, Geneva.

Kotowicz, Z. (1997) *R.D. Laing and the Paths of Anti-Psychiatry*, Routledge, London.

Laing, R.D. (1985) *Wisdom, Madness and Folly: the Making of a Psychiatrist*, Macmillan, London.

Lavalette, M. and Mooney, G. (1999) 'New Labour, new moralism: the welfare politics and ideology of "New Labour" under Blair', *International Socialism*, 2(85), pp. 27–47.

Mooney, G. (2000) 'Class and Social Policy' in Lewis, G., Gewirtz, S. and Clarke, J. (2000) *Rethinking Social Policy*, Sage, London.

Parton, N. (1991) *Governing the Family: Child Care, Child Protection and the State*, Macmillan, London.

Philo, G. (ed.) (1996) *Media and Mental Distress*, Longman, London.

Rogers, A. and Pilgrim, D. (1991) '"Pulling Down Churches": accounting for the British mental health users' movement', *Sociology of Health and Illness*, 13(2), pp. 129–148.

Rogers, A., Pilgrim, D. and Lacey, R. (1993) *Experiencing Psychiatry: Users' Views of Services*, Macmillan/MIND, London.

Sayce, L. (2000) *From Psychiatric Patient to Citizen: Overcoming Discrimination and Social Exclusion*, Macmillan, Basingstoke.

Scottish Association for Mental Health (1999) *Attitudes to Mental Health: an overview*, SAMH, Glasgow.

Sedgwick, P. (1982) *Psychopolitics*, Pluto, London.

Smith, S. (1994) 'Mistaken identity – or can identity politics liberate the oppressed?', *International Socialism*, 62, pp. 3–50.

TUC (1998) *Stress at Work*, TUC Publications, London.

Warner, R. (1994) *Recovery from Schizophrenia: Psychiatry and Political Economy*, 2nd edn, Routledge, London.

Woodward, K. (1997) *Identity and Difference*, Routledge/Open University, London.

CHAPTER 6

Deafness/Disability – problematising notions of identity, culture and structure

Mairian Scott-Hill

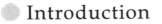 Introduction

The aim of this chapter is to examine the tension-ridden relationships between Deaf and disabled people, linking them to theoretical analyses of identity, structure and culture. On a surface level, this tension is evidenced not only by the marginalisation of Deaf people from disability politics, and *vice versa*, but also by the separate evolution of Deaf studies and disability studies. However, this chapter will examine the divisions at the deeper level of theory, taking as its basis Margaret Archer's (1996) view that the structural ('parts') and cultural ('people') domains are substantively different, as well as being relatively independent of each other. Thus theories developed about the relationship between structures and social agents and between cultures and cultural actors have to recognise the autonomy of structure and culture. The chapter argues that different theories are used in Deaf studies and disability studies to conceptualise and explain the same phenomena – identity, culture and structure. This has led to the conflation of these phenomena that has two main effects when we begin to consider the relationship between them. First, somewhat crude unilateral accounts are produced in which one of the phenomena is elided or rendered inert. Second, the phenomena are assumed to be tightly constitutive of each other, with the result that all of them disappear, and so any examination of their interconnections is precluded. Nevertheless 'parts' and 'people' are always interpenetrative, and this becomes particularly visible when their relationship is performed in the battleground of cultural politics. In this respect the structural penetration of culture in Deaf politics and the cultural penetration of structure in disability politics marks Deaf and disabled people as always already divided. In the light of this the chapter asks whether Archer's theory has limitations and concludes with a brief look at what the future might hold for political relationships between Deaf and disabled people.

Deaf studies: the structural penetration of culture

No-one disputes the fact that contemporary relationships between deaf and disabled people are fractured, nor that the meaning of the terms 'deaf' and 'deafness' are central to this. For the purpose of this chapter, I will refer to deaf people as that group of hearing-impaired people who perceive themselves to be excluded from the dominant areas of social and cultural reproduction by the perpetuation of a phonocentric world-view. They may also feel excluded from the disability movement because the movement is seen to reflect this world-view in the way in which it is socially organised around phonocentric language 'norms'. This description does not include hearing-impaired people who, with the use of hearing aids or surgically implanted devices, are able to par-ticipate fully in a phonocentric society. It does include *Deaf* people − those who use sign language and are excluded *collectively* on the basis of their status as a minority language group. Deaf people, who represent about 3−4 per cent of the larger group, include a political element that distances itself from both phonocentric society and from any suggestion that they are people with impairments or disabled people (Corker 1998). The decision to include this group in the operational definition given above is therefore immediately contested. But it should be emphasised from the outset that this definition is a *nominal* one. That is, it is not intended to signify deafness as some 'natural', innate or essential human characteristic.

From an historical perspective, much energy has been concentrated either on viewing deaf people as part of the re-articulation of a 'univer-salising discourse' on disability (Thomson 1997), or on searching for the origins of a distinct 'Deaf culture'. I will return to the first approach in the next section. For the moment, I want to begin with a focus on the search for 'culture', along with the linguistic analysis of sign language and discourse practice, which is at the heart of Deaf studies – a discipline that has evolved quite separately from disability studies. The Deaf studies agenda assumes that there must be evidence somewhere of a spontaneous and natural uprising of Deaf culture, and that conditions for this could only have been present in contexts and structures where deaf people could come together and interact socially in some form of 'community'. Language needs the social, and, in the Deaf studies view, the language in question is sign language, which is the 'natural' language of Deaf people. However, we do not know when such communities began to emerge because, as Edwards (1997, p. 31 and p. 36) notes, there were, for many centuries, formidable barriers within historical records to identifying deaf communities. For example, in societies where agriculture was the most dominant industry, or where the vast majority of the population was illiterate, deafness would not have been visible. Moreover,

> ... any condition that manifested in muteness would not have been differentiated from deafness. Muteness can result from faulty information processing brought on by forms of autism, learning disabilities and mental illness ... we are confined to learning about deafness in the ancient Greek world through the filter of the literary elite. In other words, the closest we can observe everyday life for deaf people is through the partial reconstruction of attitudes towards deaf people. Deafness was perceived not as a physical handicap but as an impairment to reasoning and basic intelligence.

What does seem to be clear is that *interpretations* of cultural discourse in particular historical contexts contrasted sharply even when the spatial and temporal location of 'culture' was the same. There is, for example, considerable documented evidence that deafness and physical impairments have been subject to very different cultural constructions at the same point and location in cultural history (Davis 1995, 1997), and this is commonly cited as one reason why Deaf and disabled people are different. For example, Winzer (1997, p. 80) notes that 'the etiology and character of deafness eluded early physicians and philosophers, the condition was usually attributed to supernatural causes. Blindness was more clearly conceptualised, and blind persons throughout the centuries generally attracted more humane treatment that did those suffering other conditions [sic].'

Nelson and Berens (1997, p. 53) comment that literary and cultural representations of deaf people 'generally begin to occur with the realisation – largely in the mid-17th century – that the deaf were actually educable in . . . the majority language of their country, and, as a result, become 'representable' *within that majority language*. It was at this point that deaf people became visible, and the term 'deaf' began to carry two meanings, one biological and the other social. As such, it seems likely that the emergence of 'Deaf culture' resulted from attempts to institutionalise particular approaches to deaf education. Wrigley (1997, pp. 54–55) says that it is therefore important to clarify who controlled this process:

> Historically, the management of Deaf identity has shifted between two contrasting but related strategies. In the traditional approach, which began with their 'discovery' by hearing people, deaf people were excluded and isolated from society as a group. Though a distinct Deaf identity was denied through removal from society, it was facilitated through this physical warehousing of deaf people together. In the modern approach, exclusion and isolation are achieved through dispersal – by mainstreaming, a watering-down of the group identity in order to deny the unintended results that isolation as a type has produced: the 'accident' of Deaf culture . . . Here again we might observe that the motivations of the conquistadors and of the 'discoverers' of Deaf people seem not so very different, nor do they seem so very different today . . . it is an open question whether today's scientific examinations seek to 'save' Deaf culture's 'soul' in order to expropriate it as an object of curiosity or they simply seek 'scientific facts'.

However, the separation of the biological and the social eventually became the basis of a distinction between biological deafness and cultural Deafness, even though Deaf people are both deaf and Deaf (Padden and Humphries 1988). Lane (1984) implies that cultural Deafness was wholly liberationary, and that sign language users were effectively rescued from the shackles of a phonocentric culture by enlightened benefactors. Therefore, the concept of 'culture' has come to rest upon the theory that the entire process of identity formation is conceived of in terms of an *optimisation framework* associated with the 'freedom' of the individual to manipulate pre-existing identities in order to achieve maximum social and material benefit (Corker 1999a). The primary motivation for this manipulation, which, it must be said, assumes that people are rational actors in this process, is the exclusion of 'negative' identity. That is, the aim is to conform to the Enlightenment ideal of the 'rational, liberal subject'. This implies that certain identities are valorised as 'positive' while others are excluded as 'negative', irrespective of the fact that 'positivity' and 'negativity' are themselves culturally constructed.

With the rise of 'modern' Deaf studies, it was *cultural* Deafness that eventually assumed the status of 'nature' within the distinction between biological deafness and cultural Deafness. Important in this respect were two things. The first was the harnessing of the knowledge that greater cultural capital is attributed to language difference than to what is perceived as pathological difference, and so sign language was increasingly promoted as the 'natural' or 'native' language of all deaf people. Indeed, Deaf people were able to see themselves as exemplars of the 'subject-of-language' approach to understanding identity, and found much support from the 'turn to language' in social theory. The second was the harnessing of the public's fascination with the 'exotic' in the pursuit of a durable 'positive' Deaf identity as 'given', which also gained much credence the rise of a 'politics of identity'. As Todorov (1993) has argued, the main exception to the tendency to regard the other as something fearful or 'negative' is the phenomenon of *exoticism*, where the other – though still misunderstood – is considered to be strange but beautiful, perhaps even superior. However, he does not view exoticism in a positive light, believing that it ranks with racism and nationalism in acting as a barrier to the acceptance of human diversity. In this respect, he says that:

> ... patriotism is the perfect mirror image of exoticism, which also forswears an absolute frame of reference but does not give up value judgments; exoticism is the opposite of patriotism in that it valorizes what does not belong to one's own country.   (1993, p. 173)

Ladd and John (1991, p. 15) suggest that 'to be involved in the political struggles [of Deaf people] gives our members the full knowledge, commitment and allegiance *of the partisan*'. The meanings of patriot and partisan are in some circumstances very similar. In the context of current moves to redefine sign language users in terms of *nation* and *nationalism*, it is probable that partisanship has evolved into some form of patriotism, as is alluded to in notions of DEAF-PRIDE and DEAF-WORLD. In this way exoticism is concerned with the valorisation of Deaf people within the majority culture whereas patriotism is part of the codification of cultural norms within the Deaf community. But, in part because of the cultural focus on belonging, solidarity and recognition, an excess of partisanship has resulted in some Deaf activists focus on rooting out the 'impurities' within their communities on the grounds of language skill, place of education, and identity 'norms' (Corker 2000a). This pits deaf people against each other as the labels assigned to alternative ways of being 'are actively policed' (Wrigley 1997, p. 225); in fact, such a view is inherent in the oft-repeated and somewhat superficial dichotomy based on the Woodward convention (1972) which translates as 'good – Deaf' and 'bad – deaf'. Put another way, cultural discourse is enmeshed in power play, and this is the main way in which structure penetrates culture.

The dichotomy between deaf and Deaf, it should be said, also implies a rejection of *impairment*, largely because its perceived 'negative' meaning appears to contradict the claim to 'naturalness' and 'nationhood' (see Corker 1998). But this only touches the surface of the complex web of linguistic interaction that constructs particular versions of impairment and disability. The sign which can be glossed as DISABILITY-OPPRESSION is a combination of the 'neutral' sign DISABLED, which does not indicate different impairments, plus the sign OPPRESSION. It is used mainly by the Deaf elite – that is, those sign language users who have been privileged in their immersion in Deaf culture and language by birthright or by educational location. And, as Wrigley (1997, p. 110) notes, paraphrasing bell hooks (1984), 'by ignoring the differences among deaf people and claiming further elite status, relatively privileged Deaf people are able to claim identification with all experience of Deafness while also assuming special authority to speak for Deaf people quite unlike themselves'. Hence, some Deaf activists, whilst using DISABILITY-OPPRESSION privately, continue to use in more public arenas the sign referred to in the British Deaf Association's BSL/English dictionary which glosses as CRIPPLE. Those who are involved in disability politics know that some disabled people use the term 'cripple' in the same way that some gays use the term 'queer' (Peters 2000). It is a political statement of defiance and pride in the face of societal oppression. But ordinary Deaf people *translate* CRIPPLE from within an understanding of disability as tragedy and pathology (Corker 2000c). Further, the meanings of 'difference' in use amongst deaf people, who are marginal to cultural politics, are by no means as clear cut, as recent work with deaf children has shown (Corker 2000c, 2001, 2004 forthcoming).

We therefore have to ask whether this use of the sign CRIPPLE is *intended* to put social distance between Deaf and disabled people. In other words, when particular sociolinguistic strategies are used by those who have 'knowledge' in the Foucauldian sense, does this amount to the strategic reinforcement of unequal power relations? Certainly, Ladd and John (1991, p. 14) argue the political position that Deaf people do not want mainstream society to restructure so that they can be included in it. Instead they must claim their inalienable 'right to exist as a linguistic minority group within that society'. In other words, linguistic minority discourses *affirm* the discourse of pathology and tragedy by emphasising their distance from it, whilst seeking to re-articulate Deaf people's 'exotic' status *within* this discourse. In a phenomenological context, then, it seems that Deaf people and disabled people represent *different* Others in their relationship with the dominant culture. Further, Ladd, writing in Jane Campbell and Mike Oliver's book *Disability Politics* (1996, pp. 120–121), suggests that it is disabled people's understanding of culture that is responsible:

> Culture as in art is one thing. Culture as in deaf culture is another. Basically, deaf people whose first language is BSL, should be seen as a linguistic minority... the whole definition of culture is so much wider than the one the disability movement is espousing. [...] The centrepiece of it is our schools... where we are socialised into the culture. Integration threatens to destroy these centres of achievement. The irony is that 80 per cent of deaf kids are integrated, with no little thanks to disabled people; we are the ones sent to the valley of Undeaf, not they.

The claim of Deaf people to particularistic minoritising rights has specific implications for contemporary relationships between Deaf people and the disability movement, because both are engaged in the pursuit of inalienable 'rights'. Further, the 'rights' in question are ultimately expressions of *contested* 'rights' to self-definition and self-determination (Shakespeare 1993; Jankowski 1997; Oliver 1996).

Disability studies: the cultural penetration of structure

It should be clear from the above discussion that *culture* is viewed by Deaf studies as the main battleground for the tension between Deaf and disabled people. On one level, this tension is explicit, as Vic Finkelstein's (1996, p. 111) rejoinder to Ladd's point about the definition of 'culture' shows:

> ... there is a great deal of uncertainty amongst disabled people whether we do want 'our own culture'. After all, we all have had experiences of resisting being treated as different, as inferior to the rest of society. So, why now, when there is much greater awareness of our desire to be fully integrated into society, do we suddenly want to go off at a tangent and start trying to promote our differences, our separate identity? Secondly, at this time, even if we do want to promote our own identity, our own culture, there has been precious little opportunity to develop a cultural life.

Later on, he describes disabled people's 'distinctive group identity' as a 'cultural' identity, and other writers refer to disability arts as 'engaging in alternative cultural production' which enables the fight back against a disabling 'culture'. However, what seems to be happening is that though two distinct meanings of culture – culture as a distinct way of life (the DEAF-WAY); and culture as the production and circulation of meaning – or 'what enables us to "make sense" of things [through] social discourses and practices which construct the world meaningfully' (du Gay et al. 1997, p. 13) – are being used interchangeably. A disability studies perspective on culture is seen to diminish Deaf people's culture.

It seems paradoxical, then, that it is the *cultural* meaning of Deafness that is reified in disability theory, but this, I suggest, is a result of the structural penetration of culture driven by a politics of identity. On one level, this contributes to the silencing of constitutive understandings of deafness because the diverse language preferences, language ability, hearing status, social identifications and personal, social and cultural identity that are as characteristic of deaf people, as they are of *any* language community are ignored (Kannapell 1993). On another level, however, for those who have little or no language of any kind, the risk of this strategy is that it can reinforce dependency on the power, administrations and benefice of the state, which defines the terms and boundaries of their lives (Corker 2000a). This likelihood significantly increases when the only social or linguistic links between separatist and mainstream cultures are *necessarily mediated by* the mainstream culture through sign language interpreters or social workers, for example. In this way, as Wrigley (1997, p. 59) notes, some deaf people have been 'appropriated and exploited for purposes entirely external to themselves [...] often ... given voices not their own. Authentic voices, in any sense of the phrase are in short supply. Signs are plentiful, but the code by which the dominant readings might be challenged is unprivileged and disenfranchised'. When the structural account is foregrounded, this amounts to disablement, which gives some weight to Finkelstein's concerns about disabled people's uncritical acceptance of the 'cultural' route to liberation, expressed quite explicitly in his work with Ossie Stuart (Finkelstein and Stuart 1996).

I am mindful, however, that more recent writing from key disability studies scholars in the UK has argued for a multi-level, multi-dimensional analysis of disability that incorporates different paradigms, along with their competing world-views and methodologies (Barnes *et al.* 1999). Indeed, writing from an American disability studies perspective, Rosemarie Garland Thomson (1997, p. 22), goes so far as to present such an analysis as a set of structures whose logical form is both *universalistic* and rooted in *structure*:

> Disability studies should become a universalizing discourse. Disability . . . would then be recognized as structuring a wide range of thought, language and perception that might not be explicitly articulated as 'disability'. I am proposing then a universalizing view of disability by showing how a concept of disability informs such national ideologies as American liberal individualism and sentimentalism, as well as African American and lesbian identities.

Such a universalist logic is presumably meant to include Deaf people – indeed Thomson does imply that this is the case on a number of occasions. But this logic clashes with the minoritising logic promoted by Deaf people, which is just one indication that its socio-cultural reception is likely to be far from universal. Indeed, when we turn the focus to disability studies, and examine how culture penetrates structure, it seems that the very way in which culture is appropriated by disability theory is part of the problem. In this context, it has to be emphasised that when tension and conflict are thought about in particular ways, this works *against* multi-level, multi-dimensional analysis. The result can be that particular world-views and methodologies are conflated and this leads to a narrowing of explanatory power rather than its broadening. Further, because ideas and knowledge are part of the *social constitution* of disability, as well as its *social determination*, and as such, they are socially embedded in the diverse realities of disabled people's lives, particular disabled people identify with and even come to signify particular ways of thinking about disability.

In Britain, disability theory as we know it emerged from and built on a document published by the Union of Physically Impaired Against

Segregation (UPIAS), called *The Fundamental Principles of Disability* (1976). The structural and material emphasis of this document on status, rights and redistribution is clear: for example, it uses the word 'social' 59 times and 'society' 24 times, but 'culture' is not mentioned at all. This document also introduces *the social model of disability*, which makes a conceptual distinction between *disability* and *impairment* – a distinction that has been and continues to be useful for explaining disability as a form of institutionalised social oppression and for challenging normative world-views. The distinction is intended, I think, as an *analytical dualism*, though it is more commonly viewed and used in practice as a *dichotomy*. This tendency to dichotomy is the subject of my earlier work, where I look at the structuration of deaf and Deaf (Corker 1998). This is because the focus on disability must be justified to a certain extent by the marginalisation of both impairment and subjectivity within a discrete analytical field. Thus impairment and subjectivity have remained under-examined *from a disability studies perspective* until comparatively recently, and even then such examination has met with strains of dis-ease (see, for example, Abberley 1987; Hughes and Paterson 1997; Corker 1998; Thomas 1999).

The tendency to use a dualism as if it were a dichotomy is also extended to the less explicit, but more fundamental distinction between structure and culture. This distinction, in connection with the relations between Deaf and disabled people, can be paralleled with Lockwood's (1964) distinction between socio-cultural integration and cultural system integration. That is, Deaf people are primarily concerned with the relationships between cultural agents, whereas disabled people are concerned with the relationships between the components of culture, and neither can be adequately analysed within a framework that conflates them. This ought not to be surprising given that the two views of culture presented above remain one of the central arguments between sociology and cultural studies (for further analysis, see Peters 2000). In this respect, and in view of Margaret Archer's concerns presented in the introduction, it is interesting that in more recent disability studies accounts, the term 'culture' has suddenly appeared *within* the structural analysis of disability. For example, Barnes *et al.* (1999, p. 2), describe disability as 'socially created' – constructed 'on top of impairment' – continuing that 'the explanation of its changing character is located in the social and economic structure and culture of the society in which it is found'. As Archer (*ibid.*) continues, 'parts' and 'people' 'are *not* co-existent through time' and so a particular structure of disability, for example, pre-dates our contemporary constitution as disabled subjects. Therefore, if 'culture' is simply 'added in', it 'prevents the interplay between "parts" and "people" from being the foundation of cultural dynamics' and so it can only underpin certain kinds of social relational models.

I want to be clear at this point that I do not dispute that disability can usefully be viewed as a social relation. However, I contest Carol Thomas' (1999, p. 40, my italics) view that an analytical approach that is focused on structure and on materialism can adequately explain disability as a product of 'social relationships *between people*'. Such analyses take a view of culture that tends to be concentrated on 'cultural system integration' (Archer 1996; *cf.* Lockwood 1964) and on 'economic reductionism' (Abberley 1998, p. 89). And, as Archer (1996, p. xvii) explains, this is perhaps a product of the pervasive 'myth of cultural integration, appropriated by sociology from early anthropology, which perpetuates an image of culture as a coherent pattern, a uniform ethos or a symbolically consistent universe'. From this perspective, 'culture is not viewed as something that is susceptible to malintegration, let alone conceptualised in terms of its degree of integration (either comparatively or historically)' (*ibid.*). I would argue that such a perspective reproduces a *specific understanding* of social relations and 'cooperation between individuals' (Marx and Engels 1970, p. 50) in the domain of 'socio-cultural integration'.

Of course, this 'image of culture' is, as we have seen, also appropriated by Deaf studies and this perhaps leads to the illusion of cultural integration, especially when it is framed by a politics of visibility. Further, like Deaf studies, disability studies extends this view of culture to a view of 'identity' as an irreducible 'given'. But this is as far as socio-cultural integration can go, because the view of language that is assumed by these images of culture and identity is often naive in that 'communication' and 'cooperation' are constructed in terms of a sender-hearer model (see Jakobson 1960). That is, a message is perceived as something that is emitted by a sender and received by a receiver, and the communicative or relational content of the message doesn't change as it circulates between human subjects. This places an emphasis on language as socially determining and sidelines its socially constitutive element, which is bound up in issues of identification and negotiation. The sender-hearer model of communication has been challenged by recent theoretical developments in communication and media studies (Luhmann 1995). It is seen to present a very limited view of the possibilities of socio-cultural integration – or to use the contemporary term 'inclusion' – in its positioning of people as mannequins who are the puppets of social structure. I feel, therefore, that this is where we begin to see signs of cultural malintegration. Thus the explanatory power of a 'social relational model' is weakened by a conflation that '*sinks* the difference between the "parts" and the "people" who hold positions or ideas within them' (Archer 1996, p. xiv).

Conclusion

As Hall (1996) suggests, the irreducibility of the concept 'identity' emerges from its centrality to the question of agency and politics. Hall uses agency in the Foucauldian (1970) sense to mean 'discursive practice', which, in Archer's terms, would threaten the relative autonomy of structure and culture. Correspondingly, Hall's interpretation brings to mind the 'subject-of-language' approach to identity, which foregrounds social constitution, and examines the unique and pervasive influence of language on human experience and activity *in socio-cultural interaction*. Thus, for Hall, politics means 'both the significance of modern forms of political movement of the signifier "identity", its pivotal relationship to a politics of location – but also the manifest difficulties and instabilities which have characteristically affected all contemporary forms of "identity politics"' (*ibid.*, p. 2).

'Identity politics' is generally taken to mean that marginalised groups generate a self-designated identity or group consciousness that is instantiated by the individual identities of its constituents. Further, some would argue that identity politics differs from many *new social movements* because the constituents of the former – such as women, gays and lesbians and people from black and ethnic minorities – are politically marked as individuals. It is also the case that claims for group rights are often a challenge to the *modern* interpretation of universal citizenship, which is itself a very powerful group identity. This is important because 'identity' is more usually viewed in its association with the cultural account, but here, it is being implied that it is also part of the structural account.

It is perhaps for this reason that, within the arena of identity, disabled people occupy a somewhat fuzzy position. First, disability is not a 'natural' category, but an elastic and transient one (Silvers 2000; Longmore and Goldberger 2000). Second, though analysis tends to present a 'politics of identity' as a 'politics of visibility', impairment is not always visible and so questions of 'marking' and 'recognition' are complex. And finally, in the global village, local actions are extremely diverse, and the clarity that can be attributed to identity becomes blurred. For example, 'identity politics' is dominant in North American approaches to analysing disability as a political question, whereas British approaches have traditionally regarded disabled people as a 'new social movement', and have favoured a 'politics of disability'. Nevertheless, though both are concerned with claiming inalienable rights, the rights in question are increasingly delineated. North American approaches (now) talk about the 'claiming' of 'knowledge and identity' that positions disabled people as cultural actors (Linton 1998), whereas British approaches emphasise the 'right' to employment, housing, transport, goods and services and so on, which positions disabled people as social agents and citizens (Oliver and Barnes 1998). Again, I must emphasise that I am talking about *dominant* trends. This is not to say that American analysis excludes 'structure' (see, for example, Russell 1998) nor that British approaches exclude 'culture' and 'identity' (see for example Shakespeare 1994; Corker and French 1999), just that these forms of analysis are elided within dominant paradigms. For disability theorists who believe the main object of struggle should be economic redistribution, cultural politics is too fragmented, incoherent and 'merely cultural' – that is too far removed from the economic realm – to achieve social transformation. To Deaf people and others, the fragmentation, incoherence and symbolism of cultural politics are precisely its political strengths. They believe that groups suffer injustices and inequalities on the basis of unequal and unfair distribution not only of economic capital but also of symbolic, social and cultural capital. Certainly, it is the latter form of capital that has assumed particular significance in the global village.

However, as Archer might suggest, perhaps the important point is that the distinction between culture and economy, cultural and structural, and hence, between redistribution and recognition is an analytical distinction that, in their everyday struggles, Deaf and disabled people do not make. Indeed, I wonder if this is the danger of analytical dualism at the level of theory because theory *itself* is located in the world of ideas and, in a dualistic relation to the world of 'people', can achieve a conflation that disembodies the world from its 'people'. In view of this, it is interesting that Archer's ideas include no more than a passing reference to the body of work that might be glossed as 'post-modern', but which includes post-structuralism, social constructionism and post-colonialism. This is in some ways regrettable because it seems to reflect the tendency within contemporary theory to draw uncritically on social and cultural metaphors that emerged at, and were contextualised by, earlier times in history. On a theoretical level, 'post-modern' work has been at the heart of the cultural penetration of structure and has informed our understanding of changing cultural, social and political structures in Western society and of the phenomenon of social constitution. One could therefore ask whether Archer's apparent suspicion of this work is yet another example of 'the fallacy of conflation', which has resulted in the erasure of troublesome theories in the dumping ground of 'post-modernism – blah, blah, blah' (Corker and Shakespeare 2002).

That being said, and particularly in view of the comments made above about people's everyday struggles, it is important to ask where

the battleground of cultural politics leaves Deaf people, and what possibilities there are for socio-cultural and cultural systemic integration. My
answer to these questions has been explored extensively in earlier work
(Corker 1998, 2000a, 2000b). Here it will be brief. From Deaf people's
perspectives, the turn to culture in disability studies should be welcome
as it might enable some interface where cultural dissonance can be
explored from a measure of common ground. It is nevertheless clear that
even in countries where a movement to cultural politics has gathered
momentum, notably North America, Deaf people are largely invisible,
except by way of anecdote, in disability studies accounts. Where Deaf
and disabled people *do* come together, it is on the basis of majority –
minority relations where they coexist rather than intermingle (Peters
2000). If there is little socio-cultural integration in reality, one has to ask
serious questions about whether Deaf people *want* to engage in disabled
people's universalistic brand of cultural politics. I think the answer to
that is negative. I also think that Deaf people's own version of cultural
politics has harnessed the support of three powerful cultural sponsors of
integration – 'exoticism', 'naturalness' and consensus with the dominant
cultural discourse – support that is sufficient to sustain its particularist
political agenda without help from disabled people. In fact, the very nature
of this sponsorship means that disabled people's involvement would be
seen as threatening. As Martha Minow (1990, p. 22) writes:

> Neither separation nor integration can eradicate the meaning of
> difference as long as the majority locates difference in a minority group
> that does not fit the world designed for the majority . . . Difference, after
> all, is a comparative term. It implies a reference: different from whom?
> And perhaps even more interesting, how much does it matter, and to
> whom?

Clearly difference matters a great deal to Deaf people (Corker 1999b,
2001). The best case scenario, then, is that disabled people's cultural
campaigns work towards a form of cultural systemic integration, which
recognises the rights of individual groups, whilst keeping in mind that
deaf people are not born *or made* equal.

References

Abberley, P. (1987) 'The concept of oppression and the development of a social
theory of disability', *Disability, Handicap and Society*, 2, pp. 5–20.

Abberley, P. (1998) 'The spectre at the feast: disabled people and social theory' in Shakespeare, T. (ed.) *The Disability Reader: Social Science Perspectives*, Cassell, London, pp. 79–93.

Archer, M.S. (1996) *Culture and Agency: The Place of Culture in Social Theory*, Cambridge University Press, revised edition, Cambridge.

Barnes, C., Mercer, G. and Shakespeare, T. (1999) *Exploring Disability: A Sociological Introduction*, Polity Press, Cambridge.

Campbell, J. and Oliver, M. (eds) (1996) *Disability Politics*, Routledge, London.

Connolly, W.E. (1991) *Identity/Difference: Democratic Negotiations of Political Paradox*, Cornell University Press, Ithaca.

Corker, M. (1998) *Deaf and Disabled or Deafness Disabled*, Open University Press, Buckingham.

Corker, M. (1999a) 'New disability discourse, the principle of optimisation and social change' in Corker, M. and French, S. (eds) *Disability Discourse*, Open University Press, Buckingham.

Corker, M. (1999b) 'Differences, conflations and foundations: the limits to "accurate" theoretical representation of disabled people's experience?' *Disability & Society*, **14**(5), pp. 627–642.

Corker, M. (2000a) 'Disability politics, language planning and inclusive social policy' *Disability & Society*, **15**(3), pp. 445–461.

Corker, M. (2000b) 'Deaf studies and disability studies: An epistemic conundrum' *Disability Studies Quarterly*, **20**(1), Winter, pp. 302–310

Corker, M. (2000c) 'Discriminatory language, talking disability, and the quiet revolution in language change' in Trappes-Lomax, H. (ed.) *Change and Continuity in Applied Linguistics*, British Studies in Applied Linguistics (15). British Association for Applied Linguistics in association with Multilingual Matters, Cleveland, pp. 115–130.

Corker, M. (2001) *Sensing Disability*, Hypatia **16**(4) (Fall), pp. 34–52.

Corker, M. (2004) *Disabled language? Analysing disability discourse as power and social practice*, Routledge, London.

Corker, M. and French, S. (1999) *Disability Discourse*, Open University Press, Buckingham.

Corker, M. and Shakespeare, T. (eds) (2002) *Disability/Postmodernity: Embodying Disability Theory*, Continuum, London.

Davis, L.J. (1995) *Enforcing Normalcy: Deafness, Disability and the Body*, Verso, London.

Davis, L.J. (1997) (ed.) *The Disability Studies Reader*, Routledge, London.

Edwards, M.L. (1997) 'Deaf and dumb in ancient Greece' in Davis, L.J. (ed.) *op.cit.*

Emanuel, J. and Ackroyd, D. (1996) 'Breaking down barriers' in Barnes, C. and Mercer, G. (eds) *Exploring the Divide: Illness and Disability*, The Disability Press, Leeds.

Finkelstein, V. (1980) *Attitudes and Disabled People: Issues for Discussion*, World Rehabilitation Fund, New York.

Finkelstein, V. (1996) in Campbell, J. and Oliver, M. (eds) *op. cit.*

Finkelstein, V. and Stuart, O. (1996) 'Developing new services' in Hales, G. (ed.) *Beyond Disability: Towards an Enabling Society*, Sage, in association with the Open University, London, pp. 170–187.

Foucault, M. (1970) *The Order of Things*, Tavistock, London.

du Gay, P., Hall, S., Janes, L., Mackay, H. and Negus, K. (1997) *Doing Cultural Studies*, Sage Publications in association with the Open University, London.

Hall, S. (1996) 'Who needs identity?' in Hall, S. and du Gay, P. (eds) *Questions of Cultural Identity*, Sage, London, pp. 1–17.

hooks, b. (1984) *Feminist Theory: From Margin to Center*, South End Press, Boston.

Hughes, W. and Paterson, K. (1997) 'The social model of disability and the disappearing body: Towards a sociology of impairment', *Disability & Society*, **12**(3), pp. 325–340.

Jakobson, R. (1960) 'Closing statement: linguistics and poetics' in Sebeok, T.A. (ed.) *Style in Language*, MIT Press, Cambridge, Mass., pp. 350–377.

Jankowski, K.A. (1997) *Deaf Empowerment: Emergence, Struggle and Rhetoric*, Gallaudet University Press, Washington.

Kannapell, B. (1993) *Language Choice – Identity Choice*, Linstok Press Inc, Burtonsville, MD.

Ladd, P. and John, M. (1991) 'Deaf people as a minority group: The political process', Block 3, Unit 9 D251, *Issues in Deafness*, The Open University, Milton Keynes.

Lane, H. (1984) *When The Mind Hears*, Random House, New York.

Linton, S. (1998) *Claiming Disability*, New York University Press, New York.

Lockwood, D. (1964) 'Social integration and system integration' in Zollschan, G.K. and Hirch, W. (eds) *Explorations in Social Change*, Houghton Mifflin, Boston.

Longmore, P.K. and Goldberger, D. (2000) 'The league of the physically handicapped and the great depression', *Journal of American History*, **87**(3), pp. 1–33.

Luhmann, N. (1995) *Social Systems*, trans. J. Bednarz, Jr., with D. Baecker, Stanford University Press, Stanford, CA.

Marx, K. and Engels, F. (1970) 'The German ideology' in Arthur, C. J. (ed.) *The German Ideology: Student's Edition*, Lawrence and Wishart, London.

Minow, M. (1990) *Making all the Difference: Inclusion, Exclusion and American Law*, Cornell University Press, Ithaca.

Nelson, J.L. and Berens, B.S. (1997) 'Spoken daggers, deaf ears and silent mouths' in L.J. Davis (ed.) *op. cit.*, pp. 52–74.

Oliver, M. (1983) *Social Work and Disabled People*, Macmillan, Basingstoke.

Oliver, M. (1990) *The Politics of Disablement*, Macmillan and St. Martin's Press, Basingstoke.

Oliver, M. (1996) *Understanding Disability: From Theory to Practice*, Macmillan, Basingstoke.

Oliver, M. and Barnes, C. (1998) *Disabled People and Social Policy*, Longman, London.

Padden, C. and Humphries, T. (1988) *Deaf in America: Voices from a Culture*, Harvard University Press, Cambridge, MA.

Peters, S. (2000) 'Is there a disability culture? A syncretisation of three possible world views', *Disability & Society*, **15**(4), pp. 583–602.

Russell, M. (1998) *Beyond Ramps: Disability after the Social Contract*, Common Courage Press, Monroe, ME.

Shakespeare, T. (1993) 'Disabled people's self-organisation: a new social movement?', *Disability, Handicap & Society*, **8**(3), pp. 249–264.

Shakespeare, T. (1994) 'Cultural representations of disabled people: dustbins for disavowal', *Disability & Society*, **9**(3), pp. 283–301.

Silvers, A. (2000) 'The unprotected: constructing disability in the context of anti-discriminatory law' in Francis, L.P. and Silvers, A. (eds) *Americans with Disabilities: Exploring Implications of the Law for Individuals and Institutions*, Routledge, New York.

Thomas, C. (1999) *Female Forms*, Open University Press, Buckingham.

Thomson, R.G. (1997) *Extraordinary Bodies: Figuring Physical Disability in American Culture and Literature*, Columbia University Press, New York.

Todorov, T. (1993) *On Human Diversity: Nationalism, Racism and Exoticism in French Thought*, Harvard University Press, Cambridge, MA.

UPIAS (1976) *The Fundamental Principles of Disability*, UPIAS, London.

Williams, G.H. *Sociolinguistics: A Sociological Critique*, Routledge, London.

Winzer, M.A. (1997) 'Disability and society before the eighteenth century' in L.J. Davis (ed.) *op. cit.*, pp. 75–109.

Woodward, J.C. (1972) 'Implications for sociolinguistic research among the Deaf', *Sign Language Studies*, **1**, pp. 1–7.

Wrigley, O. (1997) *The Politics of Deafness*, Gallaudet University Press, Washington.

CHAPTER 7

Against a politics of victimisation: disability culture and self-advocates with learning difficulties

Danny Goodley

Introduction

This chapter examines culture in the lives of people with the label of 'learning difficulties'. Drawing and building upon a recent study, it is suggested that the self-advocacy of people with 'learning difficulties' may exist prior to *and* as the consequence of joining a self-advocacy culture. Significantly, self-advocacy constitutes an alternative *cultural form* – counter to the hegemonic disabling culture – and has the potential to embrace and inform a *politics and culture of resilience*. In contrast to structuralist accounts of culture that pinpoint the victims of disabling culture, this chapter suggests that people with 'learning difficulties' display resilience that challenges victimisation. Five cultural considerations are examined. First, the embracing nature of the self-advocacy movement in terms of its potential for promoting resilient identities. Second, the role of the family in preparing members for self-advocacy. Third, the relationships between (positive) identity formation and institutionalisation. Fourth, specific disabled identities that emerge in self-advocacy culture. Fifth, the problematic though not insurmountable relationship between the self-advocacy and the disability movement. Throughout, reference will be made to the experiences and accounts of members of this counter-culture – self-advocates with 'learning difficulties'. Moreover, it will be suggested that a subtle and grounded reading of self-advocacy reveals a whole host of emerging radical cultural elements that are challenging the victimisation of people with 'learning difficulties'.

Disabling and disability cultures

The disabled activist and scholar Vic Finkelstein has recently argued that the study of culture is crucial to the development of disability studies (Finkelstein 2001). His damning view of the imminent collapse of health and welfare systems can be considered alongside the rise of new forms of professionalisation and knowledge production, raising questions about how disabled people are and can be involved in the development of a *disability culture* (see also Finkelstein and Stuart 1996):

> It is vital that all disabled people join together in their own organisation so that there is a creative interaction between disabled people who are involved with the politics of disability and disabled people involved in the arts. It is this interaction that can be particularly fruitful in helping us to take the initiative in developing a new disability culture.
>
> (Finkelstein quoted in Campbell and Oliver 1996, pp. 111–112)

Culture intertwines identities formed in political, personal, professional and private contexts. It involves cultural members acquiring knowledge to interpret and generate social and interpersonal behaviour (Spradley 1979). Crucially, culture involves *conflict*. Different levels of meaning exist within cultures that are open to reinterpretation. Historical ideas, dominant values and material expressions are constructed in such ways to include some and exclude others. Nevertheless, 'the excluded' have embraced opportunities for developing and putting in place alternatives where hegemonic culture is challenged. Giroux (1983) defines this as *resistance* to hegemonic culture. Through an analysis of youth culture, Giroux suggests that schools, clubs, streets and pubs are arenas for cultural struggle. Furthermore, within and between different cultures are acts of 'meaning-making' – what Levi-Strauss defines as *bricolage* (see Hebdige 1979). This involves the bringing together of cultural elements, which are held together by aesthetic similarity and affinity. While this may be a reassemblage of old styles, often developments in culture involve fresh ways of symbolically ordering objects and meanings to establish unique and new identities. This often involves working within but also against dominant culture.

It is possible to identify two cultural spaces inhabited by people with 'learning difficulties' in Western capitalism. The first is the dominant *disabling culture*, which posits disability and impairment as synonyms and is founded upon an individual model of disability (Oliver 1990). The dominating culture for people with 'learning difficulties' throughout the twentieth century has been one of institutionalisation and exclusion (Zetlin and Turner 1985). Policy developments in the latter part of this century appeared to challenge the cultural 'need' to exclude people so labelled from mainstream culture. Images arose of a community with open arms, welcoming back hidden lives and voices. The reality was that segregation and old attitudes persisted. In 1989 the OPCS surveys showed that 422,000 disabled people, 20 per cent of whom were below retirement age, still lived in 'communal establishments' or institutions (Martin *et al.* 1989). Across the waters, Ferguson observed that in America alone, over 125,000 people with labels of retardation remained incarcerated in large, segregated public institutions (Ferguson 1987). The hegemonic culture for disabled people has been one of exclusion, discrimination and segregation – a culture that has actively constructed the disabled person as culturally and 'socially dead' (Finkelstein 2001).

The second type of culture starting to be inhabited by people with the label of 'learning difficulties' – a *disability culture* – is grounded in the self-organisation of disabled people and has given rise to the social model of disability (Campbell and Oliver 1996; Goodley 2000). This counter-culture is testimony to the resistance of disabled people (Giroux 1983). Within this emerging disability culture, the last thirty years have brought a quiet but significant period of revolution. A politics of resilience has grown amongst people with the label of 'learning difficulties'; formally recognisable in the growth of the *self-advocacy movement*.

When many people think of self-advocacy, they think in terms of self-advocacy groups and the activities of their members. Although this perspective does not exclude the idea of individual self-advocacy, it focuses primarily on people who have consciously decided to 'speak out' or who associate themselves with groups that have taken up that standard. Hence it is possible to talk in terms of a broad movement that falls squarely in the self-help group tradition, and has strong parallels with other alliances (for example the British Coalition of Disabled People and Survivors Speak Out).   (Sutcliffe and Simons 1993, p. 36)

Self-advocacy groups are made up of members with 'learning difficulties' ('self-advocates') who attend meetings (preferably voluntarily), supported by non-disabled supporters ('advisors'). While groups are organised under a variety of names, People First is a common title. Indeed, some would suggest that People First groups constitute a self-advocacy movement in their own right (Worrell 1988). Experiences, good and bad, are divulged, opinions are shared and action taken by the group, for and with members. Previous literature on self-advocacy groups has tended to focus on constitutional and structural facets like *group type* (service-based versus independent, see Crawley 1988) and various *positions of advisors* (professionals versus volunteers, see Worrell 1988). Advisors who are professionals (care assistants, social workers, psychologists, etc.) have been attacked on the grounds that their professional accreditation, or the professionalised structures that they work within, inevitably stifle the development of self-advocacy within groups (Hanna 1978; Goodley 1997). Hence, though there has been an increase in the number of groups, this does not necessarily relate to an increase in tangible and meaningful opportunities for self-advocacy and self-determination (Crawley 1988, p. 47). Yet, a recent appraisal of self-advocacy has highlighted the resistance of self-advocates in spite of organisational tensions and broader disabling barriers (Goodley 2000). Furthermore, it could be suggested that self-advocacy contributes to the development of disability culture. These developments often involve working within and away from the dominant disabling culture.

This chapter indicates that the self-advocacy of people with 'learning difficulties' exists prior to but also as a consequence of joining the self-advocacy culture. In particular, this culture may be seen as embracing and informing a politics of resilience. Yet, in contrast to structuralist accounts of culture that pinpoint the victims of the disabling hegemonic culture, this chapter suggests that people with 'learning difficulties' are resilient and determined throughout their lives. Too often misreadings of conflict theories such as Marxism ignore the ways in which individuals challenge and resist oppression. Instead, as the early humanist Marx would suggest, labelled groups have challenged a politics of victimisation and alienation (Marx 1845).

Researching self-advocacy

This chapter draws upon and takes further a recent study of self-advocacy (Goodley 2000). First, this study involved an ethnography of four self-advocacy groups over a period of 14 months. These groups were based in a variety of service and community settings and were supported by professionals and volunteers. The aims of this ethnography were, amongst other things, to explore self-advocacy in action, to examine how self-advocates were supported and to ascertain the types of relationships groups had with health and social welfare services and other organisations (such as other organisations of disabled people). Second, the use of collaborative life story research allowed for an exploration of the impact of self-advocacy on the life experiences of a few self-advocates who have been labelled as having 'learning difficulties'. The life stories of five self-advocates, Jackie Downer, Lloyd Page, Joyce Kershaw, Anya Souza and Patrick Burke were collected. These narrators were chosen because of their extensive experience in self-advocacy groups. Issues associated with the theoretical and methodological use of narrative methods with self-advocates have been documented elsewhere (Goodley 1996, Goodley 2000). What has not been developed is an analysis of self-advocacy in relation to disability and disabling cultures. It is to this that I now turn.

Embracing cultures and resilient identities

> People First has been brilliant for me. Get up, get washed, dressed, listen to some music in the morning, go to work as normal – do what you gotta do and that's it. (Lloyd Page, in Goodley 2000, p. 85)

Self-advocacy has the potential to generate *cultural capital* – the meanings and possibilities for identity formation (see Jenkins 1992) – creating, encouraging or building further a *resilient identity*. Life stories from Goodley (2000) depict groups helping narrators to recognise, understand, clarify and develop their resilience. Patrick Burke found *People First* 'awful hard' at first because he 'didn't know what to say, how to say it or who to say it to'. He was still living in the hospital at the time and was afraid of people. Similarly, life got better for Lloyd Page when he heard of *People First*. Initially, groups provide members with opportunities to publicly recognise their voices. This is an important factor for oppressed people who are often unaware of their rights. As the Canadian self-advocate Pat Worth puts it, 'before *People First* I had no reason to live. Now I have a reason for getting up in the morning' (Yarmol 1987).

Groups can provide spaces in which to speak out to others who *listen*. Self-advocacy may be nothing new but listening often is (Worrell 1988). As Joyce Kershaw puts it: 'In *People First*, we share our problems'. Initially, this can be quite threatening, 'What you've got to look out for is they can have too much rights and all of a sudden they blow up on you' (Patrick Burke, in Goodley 2000, p. 109). Attending a place where speaking out is supported, emphasised and to which importance is attached may be a novel experience for some. Groups permitted narrators to recognise and articulate their experiences:

> You don't need to go over the top organising pictures, theatres, parties, meeting with other groups or self-help groups. Basic stuff first and campaigning later *but* you don't have to. You can just chat, you don't get the chance in the centre or at home.
>
> (Jackie Downer, in Goodley 2000, p. 82)

Groups provide a *material outlet* for self-advocacy. The confidence gained through group membership can be transferred into other contexts: 'people have changed so much' (Jackie Downer in Goodley 2000, p. 80). However, members and their groups were often engaged in a struggle for the right to 'self-advocate', as evidenced in the following vignette from one of the ethnographic research groups. Dennis, a supporter of the 'Independent group', has had confrontations with service management over his attempts to promote self-advocacy:

> Dennis told me that in addition to the Independent Group, he was supporting a Centre-based group. The members of the latter group had decided that they wanted to have their meetings outside of the Centre. They arranged to meet in a social club and Dennis told them that they were to phone if they needed him. Some days afterwards the Centre manager called Dennis into her office and demanded to know why the group had met outside, 'They could have been run over'. Dennis had replied, 'I could also have been run over – is that a problem? Should I have stayed indoors?'   (Goodley 2000, p. 163)

Interestingly, this same group developed job specifications for their supporters. The executive committee members, along with the help of other members and supporters, had prepared written documentation outlining what constituted 'a good advisor':

> A good support worker is: patient, helps people to choose, put yourself in someone else's shoes, action – to make things happen, power, where to go and let someone take risks . . . A bad support worker: doing it for other people, people who think they know best, playing god, not listening, no time to give, heart not in it, telling people what to do.
>
> (taken from the Independent Group's training notes for service staff, Goodley 2000, p. 167)

Consequently, advisors supported members in empowering ways:

> At the meeting with Norma and John from the County Council, Dennis appeared to avoid eye contact with them. When they posed questions, Dennis would look over to Robert and Andy – alerting everyone present to the two people who represented the Independent Group.
>
> (Goodley 2000, p. 167)

In this sense, then, a key cultural component of self-advocacy appears to be about emphasising the worth and value of members (over those of supporters). Members benefited from these cultural contexts – often with subtle forms of support – although a resilient identity is not solely testimony to disability culture. Indeed, these identities may be the (seemingly paradoxical) consequence of living in a disabling culture and different social groups' attempts to tackle such inequalities.

Resilience in the family

> There is, in short, a space within any oppressive social structure where human beings can operate from their own will. That autonomy may be born out of pain, or misery, out of the very forces that seek to extinguish it; but its resilience suggests the existence of a human individual separate and independent from the culture in which he operates.
>
> (Sullivan 1996, pp. 4–5)

Families of people with learning difficulties have been damned as institutions of disabled society. Koegel (1986) typifies a view of such families in which the member with learning difficulties is belittled, infantilised and cast in ways that encourage 'the retard to act as the retard'. However, in the stories of self-advocates solicited in an appraisal of self-advocacy (Goodley 2000), there appeared to be a number of childhood and adulthood experiences that occurred prior to joining self-advocacy groups that were informative in developing narrators' self-advocacy. A recurring theme for those who spoke about their family life was the determination of parents. Lloyd Page's mother had told him that there was a place for him in the world. He and his mum 'went for it'. Jackie Downer's mum was a great source of strength. Joyce Kershaw's dad was all for *People First*. Anya Souza's mother pushed for Anya to attend mainstream schools:

> In my special school everyone picked on me all the time – non-stop – either because I had Down's Syndrome or I was the odd one out. I am too bright to be in a school like that because my Mum brought me up in her natural way. To be as normal as possible.   (in Goodley 2000, p. 98)

Defiant parental figures emerge in the narratives. Systems were opposed with children. However, parents' fears can lead to tensions when children reach adulthood (Mitchell 1997, 1998). Jackie Downer and Anya Souza felt the ambivalence of being encouraged but protected by their mothers. Yet, all narrators, if they mentioned parents and family, looked back at their influence with admiration and understanding of difficulties faced. These difficulties emerge as the transition to adulthood is often hampered by dominant disabling images of 'adult with learning difficulties as child' that enter familial relationships (Koegel 1986), along with the contrasting opinions about independence held by parents and children (Zetlin and Turner 1985):

> Sometimes people with Down's Syndrome don't know about their sex lives, they don't know what it's about.
> (Anya Souza, in Goodley 2000, p. 100)
>
> Parents are very scared to let go of their children. Some parents want to do but don't know how to – always looking at the disability.
> (Jackie Downer, in Goodley 2000, p. 80)

Yet, these very difficulties appeared to *encourage dialogue* about self-advocacy. Both Anya and Jackie spoke with their mothers about their desires for independence. After separating from her husband, Joyce

Kershaw cooked and cleaned for members of her family and cared for both her ailing parents. Notions of readiness for independence appeared to have been worked through in the family. In addition, class and cultural identities are also picked up in the accounts of family ties. Following Goodley (2000), dates of birth range from the 1930s through to the 1970s. One narrator is black, one Irish and one-mixed race. Anya Souza's mother came from Prague, her father from India. Jackie Downer's cultural heritage is something she is proud of, as she thinks more and more about herself as a black woman. Joyce Kershaw reflects on the 'old days', post-war, when things were cheaper, with trips down to the local grocer's past an old woman who used to sit on the steps of her home smoking a clay pipe. The life stories pitch life as a disabled child in the web of familial identities. Consequently, disability was one of a number of identity positions held by narrators that appeared to have informed their understandings of self and others:

I had a little job in a fish and chips shop. My husband got a job as a bus conductor. Then he got a job as driver. We were married for seven years. Then he went off with my best friend. We had been friends since we were little. (Joyce Kershaw, in Goodley 2000, p. 89)

Accounts recognise that narrators' identities were not framed solely in terms of disability. By contrast, Patrick Burke mentions little about his family or background. From childhood to adulthood his home life was an institution:

I moved there in 1966. Living there was hard. I got knocked left, right and bloody centre. That's why I was afraid to speak up.
(in Goodley 2000, p. 105)

This lack of family life may partly explain why he lacked conviction in speaking up for himself prior to joining *People First*:

It really doesn't help a person's character the way the system treats you. One thing that's hard is that once you're in it, you can't convince them how smart you are . . . you're so weak you can't really fight back.
(Ed Murphy, in Bogdan and Taylor 1982, p. 218)

While families and heritage were important in developing the independence and identity of some narrators, there were times when family and self-advocacy cultures were in opposition, as evidenced in this vignette from one of the ethnographic research groups:

> Imran's father doesn't want him to come to the group. He would prefer to see him at the Centre. Dennis [the supporter] spoke with them both about how they could resolve these constraints.   (Goodley 2000, p. 169)

Mitchell's (1998) work on families has noted how the emergence in a developing culture of self-advocacy raises problematic and unanticipated issues for self-advocates and their families. Yet, families are also important in raising opportunities for dialogue – which is crucial to the development of self-advocacy. A number of other similar difficult experiences came to play a part in narrators' childhood and adulthood, as indicated in the next section.

Identity formation and institutionalisation

> I haven't had an awful lot of opportunities for work but I have done work in the past. Clearing up, dusting, and all that business. I've done household work, gardening and farm work. There used to be a farm where I lived which they're pulling down now. They're using the land for houses. It was run by a charity. They had an awful lot of farmland there and we used to look after it. There was me, Tommy, Peter, Arthur, about five or six of us. I was there for 30 years. They ran it how they wanted to run it. They didn't let you have a say about how it should be run. It was for people with learning difficulties and some of them were really bad with learning. The staff really took over – 'You can't have this, you can't have that'. It was for men like ourselves with hospital staff looking after us. The hospital staff, they could be a bit on the 'bent side' – if you know what I mean. That was a problem. They took it out on the lads who were there. That's why the majority of men don't like the hospital staff. We took them to court over a few things as well. They got fined for what they were doing. They're not running here any more. They've gone abroad, but they'll be doing exactly the same over there. I moved there in 1966.

> Living there was hard. It was very hard for me to say anything I wanted to say because if you're not big enough to fight, then you'll get a hammering. And if you're big enough to have a fight, you're all right. If you can stick up for yourself, you're okay, if you can't, then watch out. Sometimes I couldn't stick up for myself at all. Every day I was getting beaten. There was not a day missed out without me getting a good hiding. Then I would be getting raped and all that business. People don't realise it. It is true. I know it is. The people out there experiencing it, they'll tell you that it's true. Others will say it isn't.
>
> (Patrick Burke, in Goodley 2000, p. 105)

All narrators experienced institutionalisation. Lloyd Page was in day centres for 17 years. Jackie Downer was in special schools up to the age of 16. Joyce Kershaw spent her teens in a boarding school. Anya Souza spent a year in a special school against the wishes of her mother. In the hospital Patrick Burke had few mates – 'because I'd been locked up all my life'. In Goodley (2000), stories of institutions describe a continuum of exclusion. At one end institutions are boring and devaluing places, 'just sat on your backside, doing nothing'. At the other end segregation creates power inequalities that can foster sexual and physical abuse, attacking identity through psychological terrorism (Swain and French 1998). In some small way the stories like Patrick Burke's contribute to the insider literature on the history of institutionalisation:

> The telling of their experiences by people who lived for years in the large, segregated institutions has been one of the most powerful arguments for deinstitutionalisation during the past 20 years.
>
> (Ferguson et al. 1992, p. 300)

This literature has focused on the ways in which institutions endanger the development of inmates' independence. Such institutional practices threaten to erase family ties.

Narrators also reveal the *politics of diagnosis and incarceration* (contributing to other critiques such as Bogdan and Taylor 1982, Ryan and Thomas 1987 and Oliver 1990):

> My mother asked, 'Is my daughter OK?' The doctor said, 'No, she's not OK, she'll be mentally and physically handicapped for the rest of her life'.
>
> (Anya Souza, in Goodley 2000, p. 96)

> I didn't want to go but they said I had to go for my education. When I got there it seemed strange being away from home.
>
> (Joyce Kershaw, in Goodley 2000, p. 89)

In special schools, 'You were labelled as soon as you got there' (Jackie Downer, in Goodley 2000, p. 79). The impacts upon family life of former social policies are reflected on in these personal accounts. For example, Joyce Kershaw's experiences hark back to times when:

> Institutions were organised for the reception of the imbecile and idiot class of defectives who in many cases suffer from *epilepsy* and physical infirmity.   (Potts and Fido 1991, p. 11, my italics)

There is now a strong body of evidence that can be drawn upon to document the negative effects of institutionalisation, such as low self-esteem and loss of identity (e.g. Goffman 1961, 1963). People's handicaps were increased by restrictions that stifled personal development and autonomy. At its most benign, the system viewed patients as perpetual children and treated them accordingly. (Potts and Fido 1991, p. 44).

> I was stopped from speaking out. There wasn't anybody to listen to you and when I did speak out, I was shouted down.
>
> (Lloyd Page, in Goodley 2000, p. 85)

However, despite these effects of institutionalisation, self-advocates' life stories lend support to the idea that constraints have the paradoxical effect of *promoting resistance* (Fairclough 1989). Swain and French (1998) note that there are many lessons to be learnt from their accounts of disabled people that have been informed by their experiences of segregated settings. For example, narrators' scepticism about authority – or knowledge of professional culture – may be seen as a consequence of their struggles inside the system:

> Psychologists and doctors, headcases, bloody headcases they are.
>
> (Patrick Burke, in Goodley 2000, p. 110)

> The headmistress asked, 'Why is this Mongol person in my school?' I felt
> really angry, very angry.   (Anya Souza, in Goodley 2000, p. 97)
>
> I've got a bit of a negative view of doctors, nurses and professionals. You
> see, they don't listen to us.   (Lloyd Page, in Goodley 2000, p. 86)

Sceptics publicly criticise. Joyce Kershaw told the staff to call her by her surname. For all his anxieties around people, Patrick Burke remembers how he sometimes felt able to stick up for himself against the staff that abused him. Now staff are anxious when Patrick walks in the centre, 'Watch it, Paddy's here' they say. Anya Souza reprimanded a teacher for not acting when she was being bullied. Experiences of exclusion appear to equip people with a sense of injustice and ideas about good and bad practice:

> There's a lot of unemployed people who would do their job as good as
> them. We pay them. If they can't do it then that's it.
>   (Patrick Burke, in Goodley 2000, p. 108)

Those professionals that had narrators' interests at heart are remembered:

> Some professionals are ... *professionals*, others are ace – they know
> where the users are coming from.
>   (Jackie Downer, italics in original, in Goodley 2000, p. 82)
>
> A nurse said to my mother, 'Your daughter will be fine, she'll give you
> pleasure'. So I did.   (Anya Souza, in Goodley 2000, p. 96)

Joyce Kershaw was encouraged to speak up by the nurses in her school, Lesley the keyworker and the centre manager, Mr Jones. In Patrick Burke's later days in hospitals he attended an advocacy group where he formed good relationships with staff members. Finally, the life stories highlight the friendships that were made despite of the segregatory effects of institutions. Jackie Downer remembers feeling cut off from her friends when she left college. Anya still knows a lot of her peers from school. Joyce Kershaw used to play Monopoly™, cards and pool with her friends in the boarding school. Now she meets with her mates for a cup of tea in the coffee bar of the local bus station. Lloyd Page feels quite lucky having lovely neighbours. As Edgerton (1984) illustrated, while institutional cultures stress productivity, hidden and often ignored 'client subcultures' (friendship groups) emphasise sociability, harmony and the maintenance of self-esteem.

A historical overview of the disability movement demonstrates the emergence of disability cultures in and out of institutional contexts (Campbell and Oliver 1996). One of the difficult issues for disability culture is how it develops within and as an antithesis to institutional cultures. The following history of the origins of one of the ethnographic groups captures these institutional beginnings:

In 1993, Bill Shackling moved 20 miles from his home town to a group home in Cotshom. He quickly made friends with the other residents. Bill stood out, not only because of his apparent extraversion but also because of his long-standing involvement with a self-advocacy group in his old town. He was instrumental in setting up a residents' committee in this new house. By chance, two workers from a local advocacy project – John and Paul – had been in contact with Bill's old self-advocacy group. They were told that Bill had recently moved to Cotshom. The two workers were interested in developing self-advocacy links and met up with Bill soon afterwards. They offered to support a self-advocacy group that would meet separately to the residents' committee. It was not long into 1993 before the Advocacy-supported Group got off the ground, also meeting in Bill's house. Bill's experience would prove to be invaluable. He and his housemates Rudi and Guy put up posters in local Centres inviting people to join the group. Consequently a number of new members joined, including residents from a local 'autistic community'. Before long, some members from the original residents' committee who had joined at the start had now left, so a new venue was sought. Bill, Rudi and Guy looked over a number of places before plumping for the Youth Club, handily located just down the road from their home.

(Goodley 2000, pp. 155–156)

Levine and Langness (1986) have argued that people with 'learning difficulties' tend to lead marginal existences. They do not reside contiguously nor even necessarily interface with one another and do not consciously share any common identity or a wish to do so. This argument reflects a view of institutions as structurally constraining residents in such ways as to deny them a culture. However, life stories of self-advocates point to the resilience that may be fostered in these deculturising places that actually sows the seeds for the production of a counter-culture, including perceptive critiques of professionalisation and the development of alternatives, most notably via self-advocacy.

Disabled identities and self-advocacy culture

Throughout my involvement with self-advocacy groups, one of the key recurring concerns for people with learning difficulties is their problematic relationship with notions of 'disability', 'impairment' and 'learning difficulties'. Gillman *et al.* (1997) suggest that the culture of the self-advocacy movement deals with notions of normality and disabled identities in very different ways to the wider disability movement. While physically impaired activists have challenged the medicalisation of their bodies through a re-appropriation of the 'disabled body' discourse (as exhibited through slogans such as 'disabled and proud'), the self-advocacy movement has tended to both use and refuse the label of learning difficulties (hence the adoption of 'People First' by many self-advocacy groups). It is possible to speculate on three cultural reactions to the label within the self-advocacy movement. First, 'learning difficulties' is embraced as a far more positive label than previous terms such as 'mental retardation' in order to recognise intrinsic and individual difference and variability:

> We are people with learning difficulties, not what people used to call us. I won't say the word. (Joyce Kershaw, in Goodley 2000, p. 230)
>
> Learning difficulties is more dignified.
> (Jackie Downer, in Goodley 2000, p. 81)
>
> Mental impairment? Now what the hell's that? Never heard of it. I've heard of learning disability. I think mental handicap is still being used but they shouldn't. (Patrick Burke, in Goodley 2000, p. 109)
>
> Who has 47 cells? I have. They haven't they've only got 46.
> (Anya Souza, in Goodley 2000, p. 99)

Second, labels are there to be rejected. After all, 'learning difficulties' means abnormal and is hardly something to be positively embraced:

> Would I say I have difficulties learning? No, I learnt well enough. I picked up things very quickly ... You can't say you're 'just handicapped' because you're labelling someone and that's not the way to talk to someone.   (Anya Souza, in Goodley 2000, p. 101)
>
> 'Learning disabilities' – I don't like that, disability makes you believe that we are in wheelchairs and we can't do anything for ourselves, when we can. We've got jobs now, we've got paid jobs.
>   (Joyce Kershaw, in Goodley 2000, p. 229)

Third, and perhaps most interestingly, 'learning difficulties' is opened up for wider analysis – as something to be adopted or applied to oneself, others or, indeed, anyone:

> A man couldn't do woman's work ... I said, 'You want to come and see some of them working in the centre and I bet they'd have to teach you how to do it'. Come and try and do our work and you'll soon find out if you've got a learning difficulty or not.
>   (Joyce Kershaw, in Goodley 2000, p. 230)

The existence of these different positions suggests that self-advocacy groups provide a cultural space for destabilising naturalised notions of impairment (Goodley 2001). Indeed, we could argue that groups allow a context for bricolage: of using old symbols and signs and turning them around to invent new cultural forms. This is crucial to self-advocacy culture. In many cases, self-advocacy groups provide safe discursive places for revamping, experimenting, rejecting and adopting terminology which is utilised to create identities. This raises two concerns in relation to identity and cultural discourses. First is the issue of 'impairment-specific' identities. Much of the British disability studies literature rejects specific impairment groupings on the basis that such distinctions disrupt the common ground of a disability culture through a classic individualistic focus on bodily and psychological difference (Oliver 1990; Barnes *et al.* 1999). While such a rejectionist position is understandable in view of the meddling by 'impairment-specific' charities and organisations *for* disabled people in the lives of disabled people, we must be careful not to ignore the ways in which self-advocacy cultures deal directly with the 'impairment-specific' nature of being labelled as having 'learning difficulties'. The self-advocacy movement does not simply reconstitute impairment-specific concerns within the wider disabled people's movement but engages with the ways in which the specific meanings of particular labels threaten the very humanity of activists. As noted above, one strategy adopted is to open up wider meanings of 'learning difficulties' and pitch them in a variety of contexts and life experiences ('a man couldn't do woman's work', Joyce Kershaw). Whether or not we agree with the sentiments of such deconstructive tactics, self-advocacy appears to have the potential to disrupt 'learning difficulties' in ways that align it with other contemporary examples of 'identity politics' (see Parker and Shotter 1990). Current British cultural forms and political activities are evidently engaged with analyses of the artefacts of the 'knowledge society' (see Bell 1973; Jameson 1984). A consequence of such analyses could be a view of such phenomena as 'learning difficulties' as transient, cultural and ever-changing in contrast to the traditional view of 'impairments' as permanent, natural and static entities. Here, we have a key characteristic of new social movements at play: the making of a strong ideological shift in thinking about oneself (see Shakespeare 1993; Boggs 1996).

Second, is the issue of defining someone as a 'self-advocate'. Just as soon as people with learning difficulties are speaking up for themselves, then another (pseudo-professionalised) term is lying in wait to be applied. 'Otherness' is emphasised, people with 'learning difficulties' are seen as only exhibiting the 'skills of self-advocacy' in self-advocacy groups (never outside) and, most importantly, they are now 'self-advocates' rather than 'disabled activists'. It has been argued elsewhere (see Goodley and Moore 2001), that the actions of people who have been labelled as having learning difficulties need to be recognised, publicised and theorised in order to truly characterise their activism. In many cases in self-advocacy groups this may take place at the very personal level of human rights but should be viewed as activism nonetheless:

Sarb is having problems at home. His brother picks on him and tells him what to do. Karen agreed, she hates it when staff watch her having a bath.
(Goodley 2000, p. 192)

Karen had recently had a meeting with an educational psychologist because, she joked, 'I'm dumb in the head'. A supporter who works at the college suggested that this meeting be arranged because Karen 'was not joining in in class'. Karen disagreed – 'No, I were bored'.
(Goodley 2000, p. 191)

'I used to be a member of loads of committees fighting for rights and all that ... yeah, and the Disability Movement do some great stuff for other people, but how's all that stuff on politics going to get me a girlfriend and a job?'
(Tiger Harris, life story, from Armstrong and Goodley 2001, p. 9)

These vignettes present members of self-advocacy groups resiliently seeking basic human rights – personal privacy, refuting others' presumptions and seeking a partner – all emphasising adult roles (Mitchell 1998). For people with 'learning difficulties', the most basic rights are denied so often but there is a danger that we lose sight of them as we get caught up in the changing elements of policy and welfare (Means and Smith 1994). In some ways then, perhaps the culture of self-advocacy necessitates a view of disability politics that is sensitive to the private and political agendas of (disabled) people (with learning difficulties), as well as the public and political agendas of the movement. These wider concerns with the movement are taken further in the next section.

● Self-advocacy and the disability movement

It is no small challenge to the movement to ensure that barriers are eradicated so that no impaired group is disadvantaged.

(Campbell and Oliver 1996, p. 96)

Any analysis of disability culture necessitates a consideration of the disabled people's movement. Briefly, I want to explore three areas in relation to self-advocacy and the wider disabled people's movement. First, let us consider the issue of separate movements. Much of the literature by and on self-advocacy groups has noted the difficulties involved in making links with the wider disability movement. Misgivings include the potential of articulate physically impaired activists to dominate the agenda (Chappell 1998) and the under-representation of people with 'learning difficulties' in coalitions of disabled people (Simons 1992). Barnes *et al.* (2000) found that Centres for Independent Living in Britain under-represented people with learning difficulties particularly in the early years of an organisation's life. Interestingly, in my research, one self-advocacy group – the 'Independent Group' – saw their increasing independence from the local Council for Integrated Living and Council of Disabled People as a positive development. For them becoming a 'real' self-advocacy group was about becoming independent of other groups' involvement – whether they were organisations of or for disabled people. Here, perhaps, we have something fundamentally specific to the activism of a self-advocacy culture: that collective (and individual) organisation is about displaying independence and capability. More about this later.

Second, we need to pay attention to the role of professionals in self-advocacy groups. The involvement of advisors or supporters in self-advocacy groups blurs a typical British disability studies distinction between organisations of and for disabled people. Oliver's (1990) typology of organisations makes the case for the increasing politicisation of disabled people as they move from organisations *for* (including partnership with and patronage by parental, professional or parliamentarian bodies) to organisations *of* (with consumerist, self-help, populist and activist leanings connected by umbrella and coordinating bodies). This increasing politicisation (and independence) of disabled people involves a corresponding decrease in the professionalisation (and dependency) of organisations of disabled people. For Oliver (1990, 1996) when professionals become involved in organisations of disabled people, ambitions associated with career advancement and an uncritical acceptance of the individual model of disability threaten the interdependence of disabled activists. However, a typology that views professional involvement as undermining the activism of disabled people has massive implications if applied to an analysis of the self-advocacy movement. Indeed, my ethnography of self-advocacy groups suggests that it is not professional involvement *per se* that limits or enables self-advocacy but the nature of interventions made by supporters in groups. As I have documented elsewhere (Goodley 1997, 1998, 2000) supporters appear to draw upon a variety of discourses associated with such notions as 'deficit' and 'capacity' that, respectively, demote or promote the self-determination of self-advocacy groups. This in itself has consequences for the ways in which supporters view their own roles and commitment to the tenets of self-advocacy. The following narrative from ongoing research (see Armstrong and Goodley 2001) displays the complexities of supporting:

Another day for Paul, a care assistant and supporter of the self-advocacy group based in Forest House, a MENCAP-supported group home for five adults with learning difficulties. Another day of watching TV chosen by residents, of making tea and coffee if residents allowed, of washing clothes and bed sheets after lengthy discussions with two residents who like to do their own washing. As we sat together in the kitchen, late afternoon, over a cup of tea, Paul reflected aloud, 'This is meant to be the way you support self-advocacy, isn't it? Good support is not doing anything. But why am I here?'

To present professionals as unreflective purveyors of dependency and oppression is a structuralist conclusion often made in disability

studies literature. Nevertheless, regardless of how enabling professionals and supporters are, an argument remains that the very existence
of professional/advisor–client/self-advocate relationships still leaves
spaces for the emergence of a professional culture (organisations *for*)
instead of a disability culture (organisations *of*). Shakespeare (2000)
offers an alternative vision by drawing upon a feminist ethics of care. He
argues that the tendency in disability studies to separate 'care' (which
entails professional involvement and the creation of dependency) from
'justice' (associated with disability politics and the development of
independence) is a classic modernist mistake. To view neediness for care
or support as a threat to autonomy promotes the view that more needy
people are, therefore, less autonomous – a stereotype that disabled
people are used to challenging. To view support or care as the stuff of
dependency ignores the fact that any political, personal or cultural act
relies upon the support of others, it is an integral part of human existence. We need to recognise that we are all vulnerable, dependent and
finite and that we all have to find ways of dealing with this in our daily
existence. Care and support are not just things that disabled people
need. Yet the dominance of liberal traditions of independence and individualism – that emphasise the voluntary and rational components
of the human condition – ignores the ways in which we are all always
constructed relationally. We need to analyse disability cultures in terms
of a:

> community of selves . . . in a certain culture and epoch of history, i.e. an
> embedded self. Hence, the possibility of self-hood, agency, personal
> autonomy, universalism and so forth, is reinterpreted in light of this
> expanded identity.   (Reindall 1999)

Consequently, typologies of organisations *of* and *for* disabled people
may not only set up straw men but may ignore the occurrence of interdependence between non-disabled and disabled people in the politics of
disabled people. Interestingly, more and more organisations for disabled
people are being represented by disabled people. Disabled people's
representation on RADAR's management committee is now 51 per cent
(Morgan 2001). However, critical questions remain as to the extent
of meaningful involvement and commitments to interdependence. As
Morgan (2001) notes, the disabled people's movement needs to define
what is meant by a user-led organisation of disabled people. Does it
need to be more than numerical dominance on management committees? Should it involve a commitment to social model principles? This

leads me to the third and last issue raised in my research: the bureau-cratisation of self-advocacy. Evidently, the success of the self-advocacy movement has been reflected in the growth of independent self-advocacy groups that function independently of services, are well funded through lottery and other funding initiatives, with independent and accountable advisors, providing members with daily experiences for working as self-advocates. One such group is the Independent Group:

The Independent Group is an innovative, independent self-advocacy project based in Blaketon. The project is run and managed by people with a learning difficulty, supported by three part-time workers. There are only a handful like it in the country. The main aim of the group is to support adults with learning difficulties in speaking out, making choices and decisions, becoming aware of their rights and to manage the Independent Group themselves. In early 1992 a group of people got together to form a steering group to set up the Independent Group – five people with a learning difficulty, a member of Blaketon Coalition for Disabled People, a person who worked for MENCAP and two people from Blaketonshire Centre for Integrated Living (BCIL) who were holding the money obtained from voluntary services. The steering group drew up a person specification for the job of project support worker, interviews were held and presentations given. Members with learning difficulties on the interview panel could not separate two people. They suggested a job share. They [Dennis and Julia] agreed and started in late 1992. By mid-1993 there were ten new members meeting in Blaketon every Thursday. The group provided a training day on making information accessible to non-readers and soon after acquired their own office space in a community building. Computer, phone, copier, fax, TV, video, camcorder and kettle were all acquired. They became active in the Blaketon Coalition of Disabled People to show what things are important to people with learning difficulties and continued to carry out training days on 'self-advocacy' and related issues for service users, students and staff. Presently . . . 20 people are involved in the project.

(Official introductory leaflet obtained at first meeting, from Goodley 2000, p. 162)

Groups such as this provide possible employment opportunities as well as an alternative to Day Centres and sheltered workplaces. Such opportunities take on a salient character in the light of the inadequacy of the Disability Discrimination Act (1995) for promoting real work for disabled people (see Barnes 1996). This group demonstrates the involvement of disabled people in training policy-makers, professionals and carers in disability rights and self-advocacy. Still, questions are also raised about the purpose of such groups (self-help, training of service staff, politicisation of people with learning difficulties and so on). Indeed, as Page and Aspis (1997) have argued, major question marks remain in relation to the (in)voluntary nature of membership of a self-advocacy culture. They note that if self-advocacy becomes yet another service provision (part of the curricula of day centres, a section of a syllabus on a 'social skills' course at the local college) or, indeed, an alternative to services (as in the case, potentially, of the 'Independent Group') then there are dangers that self-advocacy will be hijacked. Training of service staff will take priority over members' own development. Furthermore, a commitment to the bureaucratisation of self-advocacy may take precedence over informal though significant cultural elements of activism. I have spoken about this elsewhere in terms of 'contextualised activism' (see Goodley and Moore 2001) – where people engage in microscopic interactions that might not fit with the public, macro and campaigning forms of activism so celebrated by new social movements but which are resistant nonetheless:

> It's helped me being in a self-advocacy group because my friends help me to stick up for myself. When my friends are down, I help them and when I am down, they help me.
>   (Dorna Mack, life story, from Armstrong and Goodley 2001, p. 13)

Conclusion

This chapter has highlighted the ways in which resilience occurs in spite of disabling practices and as a consequence of a developing culture of self-advocacy. It has made a case for self-advocacy as resilience and has challenged the assumption that the identity of 'learning difficulties' is one tied to victimhood. Reflecting on the stories of 'fit people who were removed' into institutions, Potts and Fido (1991, p. 139) concluded:

> That side by side with a painful awareness of lost lives, we have also become sensitive to their humour, resilience and determination. Far from accepting their lot in life, they recognise its injustices and have eagerly grasped the opportunity to give their view of The Park and its history.

Following Goodley (2000: 200–02) a number of things appear to characterise resilience. First, it is *contextualised*, looming in a variety of sociopolitical and inter-relational contexts. Families, professionals, schools and work influence and shape its emergence. For some, the very experience of disablement appears to inform their subsequent resilience. For others, inclusive relationships with family and professionals were necessary in encouraging self-determination. When Marx (1832) wrote in *The German Ideology* that 'life determines consciousness', he was aware of the contradictory social conditions of oppression and resistance from which comes forth sensuous awareness of individuality and society. Later, in *Theses on Feuerbach* (1845), he observed that human essence is 'the ensemble of social relations . . . [belonging] to a particular form of society'. Similarly, self-advocacy groups have the potential to invite the development of a consciousness that is sensitised to disabling *and* enabling conditions from which resilience emerges. In this sense, then, resilience allows us some explanatory value in assessing the impact of social contexts upon people with 'learning difficulties'. The doing of self-advocacy may provide access to social networks that help resilience to germinate from potential to action. In this sense, then, resilience seems to reside in the space between structure and individuality. It is not an individual attribute or a structural product. Hence, and secondly, resilience is *complicating*. It is anti-essentialist as it troubles notions of naturalised impairment and is against crude-structuralist takes on disablement. It appears to be associated with the mid-ground of theorising social life, flirting with notions of pre-existing potential for personal and collective resistance while locating understandings in social contexts. Third, it is *optimistic*. It is related to the capacity of human nature to resist oppression, challenging the tendency to underestimate people with the label of 'learning difficulties'. Resilience as a phenomenon questions how we understand the concept of 'learning difficulties'. There is a need for supporters, professionals, researchers and policymakers to assume the potential for resilient lives when developing collaborative work with people with 'learning difficulties'. Fourth, it is *interpersonal*, open to various forms of intervention and social interaction, highlighting the support of others that enables or denies. Finally, resilience is *indicative of disablement*. Alongside shows of resistance, this chapter has revealed stories and observational vignettes of disabling ideologies, environments, attitudes and actions that permeate the lives of self-advocates. There is a danger of romanticising the 'autonomy' of self-advocates if we ignore their day-to-day experiences of oppression. Self-advocacy groups appear to provide a place in which self-advocacy can potentially be supported. For some people, like Patrick Burke, joining a group is instrumental in recognising and developing self-determination, from damaging environments to embracing groups. Other members of self-advocacy made similar points about the changes that occurred for them when they joined their group, 'We were allowed to speak our minds' (Goodley 2000, pp. 201–202). In the final analysis, a study of disability culture needs to be aware of the subtle, personalised and often microscopic elements of activism. One such way is to embrace and theorise resilience whilst challenging analyses that may actually recreate victims of disablement.

References

Armstrong, D. and Goodley, D. (2001) *Self-advocacy, Civil Rights and the Social Model of Disability: Final Report to the ESRC* (Research Grant R000237697). University of Sheffield, Sheffield.

Barnes, C. (1996) *What Next? Disability, the 1995 Disability Discrimination Act and the Campaign for Disabled Peoples' Rights*, paper presented at the Walter Lessing Lecture (Part 2) Skill (National Bureau for Disabled Students) Annual Conference, London.

Barnes, C., Mercer, G. and Shakespeare, T. (1999) *Exploring Disability: A Sociological Introduction*, Polity Press, London.

Barnes, C., Mercer, G. and Morgan, H. (2000) 'Creating independent futures: An Evaluation of Services Led by Disabled People: Stage One Report', University of Leeds Press, Leeds.

Bell, D. (1973) *The Coming of Post-industrial Society*, Heinemann, London.

Bogdan, R. and Taylor, S. (1982) *Inside Out: The Social Meaning of Mental Retardation*, University of Toronto Press, Toronto.

Boggs, C. (1996) *Social movements and Political Power*, Temple University Press, Philadelphia.

Campbell, J. and Oliver, M. (1996) *Disability Politics: Understanding our Past, Changing our future*, Routledge, London.

Chappell, A. (1998) 'Still Out in the Cold: People with Learning Difficulties and the Social Model of Disability' in T. Shakespeare (ed.) *The Disability Reader: Social Science Perspectives*, Cassell, London.

Crawley, B. (1988) *The Growing Voice: A Survey of Self-advocacy Groups in Adult Training Centres and Hospitals in Great Britain*, Values into Action, London.

Edgerton, R.B. (1984) 'The Participant-Observer Approach to Research in Mental Retardation', *American Journal of Mental Deficiency*, 88(5), pp. 498–505.

Fairclough, N. (1989) *Language & Power*, Longman, London.

Ferguson, P. (1987) 'The Social Construction of Mental Retardation', *Social Policy*, 18, pp. 51–56.

Ferguson, P.M., Ferguson, D.L. and Taylor, S.J. (1992) 'Introduction' in Ferguson, P.M., Ferguson, D.L. and Taylor, S.J. (ed.) *Interpreting Disability: A Qualitative Reader*, Teachers College Press, New York.

Finkelstein, V. (2001) *A Personal Journey into Disability Politics*. Paper presented to the Leeds University Centre for Disability Studies as part of 'New Directions in Disability Seminar Series', 7th February.

Finkelstein, V. and Stuart, O. (1996) 'Developing New Services' in Hales, G. (ed.) *Beyond Disability: Towards an Enabling Society*, Sage/Open University Press, London.

Gillman, M., Swain, J. and Heyman, B. (1997) 'Life History or "Care History": The Objectification of People with Learning Difficulties through the Tyranny of Professional Discourses', *Disability and Society*, **12**(5), pp. 675–694.

Giroux, H. (1983) *Theory and Resistance in Education*, Bergin and Havey, New York.

Goffman, E. (1961) *Asylums*, Doubleday, New York.

Goffman, E. (1963) *Stigma: Some Notes on the Management of Spoiled Identity*, Penguin, Harmondsworth.

Goodley, D. (1996) 'Tales of Hidden Lives: A Critical Examination of Life History Research with People who have Learning Difficulties', *Disability and Society*, **11**(3), pp. 333–348.

Goodley, D. (1997) 'Locating Self-advocacy in Models of Disability: Understanding Disability in the Support of Self-advocates with Learning Difficulties', *Disability and Society*, **12**(3), pp. 367–379.

Goodley, D. (1998) 'Supporting People with Learning Difficulties in Self-advocacy Groups and Models of Disability', *Health and Social Care in the Community*, **6**(5), pp. 438–446.

Goodley, D. (2000) *Self-advocacy in the Lives of People with Learning Difficulties: The Politics of Resilience*, The Open University Press, Buckingham.

Goodley, D. (2001) '"Learning Difficulties", the social model of disability and impairment: challenging epistemologies', *Disability & Society*, **16**(2), pp. 207–231.

Goodley, D. and Moore, M. (2001) 'Doing Disability Research: Activist Lives and the Academy', *Disability and Society*, **15**(6), pp. 861–882.

Hanna, J. (1978) 'Advisor's Role in Self-Advocacy Groups', *American Rehabilitation*, **4**(2), pp. 31–32.

Hebdige, D. (1979) *Subculture: The meaning of style*, Methuen, New York.

Jameson, F. (1984) 'Postmodernism, or the cultural logic of late capitalism', *New Left Review*, 146.

Jenkins, R. (1992) *Pierre Bourdieu*, Routledge, London.

Koegel, P. (1986) 'You Are What You Drink: Evidence of Socialised Incompetence in the Life of a Mildly Retarded Adult' in Langness, L.L. and Levine, H.G. (eds) *Culture and Retardation*, D. Reidel Publishing Company, Kluwer.

Levine, H.G. and Langness, L.L. (1986) 'Conclusions: Themes in an Anthropology of Mild Mental Retardation' in Langness, L.L. and Levine, H.G. (eds) *Culture and Retardation*, D. Reidel Publishing Company, Kluwer.

Martin, J., White, A. and Meltzer, H. (1989) *Disabled Adults: Services, Transport and Employment*, OPCS, London.

Marx, M. and Engels, F. (1932/1962) *The German Ideology*, Progress Publishers, Moscow.

Marx, K. (1845) 'Theses on Feuerbach' in Marx, K. and Engels, F. (eds) *Selected Works*, Lawrence & Wishart, London.

Means, R. and Smith, R. (1994) *Community Care: Policy and Practice*, Macmillan, Basingstoke.

Mitchell, P. (1997) 'The Impact of Self-advocacy on Families', *Disability & Society*, 12(1), pp. 43–56.

Mitchell, P. (1998) *Self-advocacy and Families*, Unpublished PhD Thesis, Open University.

Morgan, H. (2001) 'Creating Independent Futures: Preliminary Findings', Presentation to the Surrey Users Network, Burpham, Surrey, 22/11/01.

Oliver, M. (1990) *The Politics of Disablement*, Macmillan, Basingstoke.

Oliver, M. (1996) *Understanding Disability: From Theory to Practice*, Macmillan, London.

Page, L. and Aspis, S. (1997, Dec 1996/ Jan 1997) Special feature. *Viewpoint*, pp. 6–7.

Parker, I. and Shotter, J. (eds) (1990) *Deconstructing Social Psychology*, Routledge, London.

Potts, M. and Fido, R. (1991) *A Fit Person to be Removed: Personal Accounts of Life in a Mental Deficiency Institution*, Northcote House, Plymouth.

Reindall, S.M. (1999) 'Independence, Dependence, Interdependence: Some Reflections on the Subject and Personal Autonomy', *Disability & Society*, 14(3), pp. 353–367.

Ryan, J. and Thomas, F. (1980 and 1987) *The Politics of Mental Handicap*, revised edn 1987, Free Association Press, London.

Shakespeare, T. (1993) 'Disabled People's Self-organisation: A New Social Movement?', *Disability, Handicap and Society*, 8(3), pp. 249–268.

Shakespeare, T. (2000) *Help*, Venture Press, Birmingham.

Simons, K. (1992) *'Sticking Up For Yourself': Self Advocacy and People with Learning Difficulties*, Community Care Publication in Association with The Joseph Rowntree Foundation.

Spradley, J.P. (1979) *The Ethnographic Interview*, Holt, Rinehart & Wilson, New York.

Sullivan, A. (1996) *Virtually Normal: An Argument About Homosexuality*, Vintage Books, London.

Sutcliffe, J. and Simons, K. (1993) *Self-advocacy and Adults with Learning Difficulties: Contexts & Debates*, The National Institute of Adult Continuing Education in association with The Open University Press, Leicester.

Swain, J. and French, S. (1998) *Lessons from Segregation*, paper presented at the Policy, Failure and Difference Seminar, Ranmoor Hall, Sheffield.

Taylor, S.J. and Bogdan, R. (1989) 'On Accepting Relationships between People with Mental Retardation and Non-disabled People: Towards an Understanding of Acceptance', *Disability, Handicap & Society*, 4(1), pp. 21–37.

Worrell, B. (1988) *People First: Advice for Advisors*, National People First Project, Ontario, Canada.

Yarmol, K. (1987) 'Pat Worth – Self-Advocate par excellence', *Entourage*, 2(2), pp. 26–29.

Zetlin, A.G. and Turner, J.L. (1985) 'Transition from Adolescence to Adulthood: Perspectives of Mentally Retarded Individuals and their Families', *American Journal of Mental Deficiency*, 89(6), p. 570.

CHAPTER 8

Now I Know Why Disability Art Is Drowning in the River Lethe (with thanks to Pierre Bourdieu)

Paul Anthony Darke

Introduction

I start this chapter by giving an overview of Disability Arts as it is now and compare this with what it initially could have been. I will also make some comments on the reality of funding and what funders' actual aims are for Disability Art. I then move on to the ideas of Pierre Bourdieu, linking them directly to Disability Arts, to show how and why Disability Art has been negated as a potentially significant art practice in contemporary art culture in the UK (and, most likely, in other cultures as well). I argue that Disability Art has had such significance because it has the potential, as we will see, to deconstruct the images which society creates through its art and other hegemonies of normality. Such hegemonies legitimise society's own sense of what is 'good' art, a 'normal' body and a 'vibrant' culture.

The development of Disability Art in the UK

Disability Art was first a significant item on the agenda of disability politics between 1985 and 1987, a period during which the London

Disability Arts Forum was founded along with its seminal Disability Arts magazine DAIL. The even glossier Disability Arts Magazine (DAM) followed a few years later. Disability Arts had been around before in the UK, and in the USA, but for Britain the mid-1980s was the beginning of a Disability Arts culture linked to and coming from within the political disability movement of the 1970s and 1980s. Great hopes, combined with immense excitement, were held by all involved; it would be a truly inclusive, accessible, revolutionary and egalitarian cultural expression in a mainstream culture which excluded, discriminated, used and abused disabled people both culturally and in its own social and artistic fantasies (Campbell and Oliver 1996; Morrison 1990). Disability Art used art to identify and reveal how 'cultural forms and practices do not simply reflect an already given social world but, rather, play a constitutive role in the construction of that world' (Bowler 1994). In this respect Disability Art saw, from its inception, that the art establishment, through its exclusion of disabled people and its continuing denial of disability as a social issue, played an important role in the social and cultural exclusion of disabled people.

Thus, Disability Art philosophy is based upon legitimising the experience of disabled people as equal within art and all other cultural practices. Disability Art is not to be seen as an equal opportunities issue but as part of a process of re-presenting a more accurate picture of society, life, disability and impairment and art itself. Disability Art is a challenge to, an undermining of (as a minimum), traditional aesthetic and social values. Coming out of post-1960s liberal ideas of social and material constructivism, Disability Art is virtually a sociology of the art of society. Art is used to explore its own disabling practices and processes. Disability Art utilises the social model of disability (and society) to explore disability (not impairment *per se*) and society through arts practice and culture as a collective and individual experience of socio-economic exclusion in a society that is marginalising, demeaning and exploitative of the images and experience of disabled people.

Disability Art is about the nature of the barbarism of contemporary culture in relation to itself through explorations of the construction of otherness and disability. As most non-disability canonical art practice was, and still is, structured around the cultural hegemonic of normality, Disability Art is a threat to the core aesthetic values of contemporary cultures. Thus, Disability Art is, perhaps, the last great revolutionary art at humanity's disposal that is solely humanitarian and non-ideological in intent. The transformative potential of the Disability Arts movement was recognised by Oliver (1990) who commented:

> The disability arts movement is increasingly becoming the focus of the mounting of these challenges (against dominant disablist imagery) but it has, itself, had to struggle to free itself from the domination of able-bodied professionals who tended to stress art as therapy (Lord 1981) rather than art as cultural imagery. That, too, is changing as disabled people struggle to take control of their lives.   (Oliver 1990, p. 62)

The problem is that you will almost never see any actual Disability Art in a theatre, museum, gallery or even at a Disability Arts festival. Even if you do, it is there because it has been mis- or re-interpreted. Mostly, though, what you will see is pseudo-therapy workshop products or impairment-orientated works. Usually it will be from a craft basis or developed in an empowerment course, superficially structured within the social model of disability but actually impairment-specific. This might be described as low level Community Arts. Alternatively, you will see workshops being done to fulfil a Lottery application or other funding body's equal opportunities prerequisite. Worse still, you will see works that are rooted in the conventional norms of society: 'heroic works' that assert the potential normality of disabled people to fit in (for example, Candoco, Chicken Shed Theatre, Heat and Soul, Blue Eyed Soul and the like). Non-disabled people love this 'overcoming their disabilities' kind of performance, 'activities' which triumph the ideals of the 'normal' through parody or pastiche. Such art 'activities' have nothing to do with Disability Art, but they are to do with traditional preconceptions of art or therapy or, worse, as some form of inspirational role modelling. The aim of this chapter is to reveal the changing relationship between cultural ideas (Disability Art) and the processes and practices of cultural institutions – specifically, the art establishment. It is only in doing this that we can see where we actually set out from and, more significantly, why we did not get where we wanted to go.

If the function of culture (specifically that part of culture called art) is to encourage the cultural museums (galleries, art schools, venues and the like) to legitimise the hegemony of normality (Bourdieu 1993) and reinforce the otherness of disabled people, then a re-evaluation of Disability Art is overdue. Such a re-evaluation is particularly relevant, given the growth of cultural homogenisation and the increasing alienation and exclusion of disabled people from the broader elements of cultural life. Practices such as genetic screening, the 'statementing' of disabled children in schools and the 'sectioning' of people with mental health problems in the community all emphasise the otherness of disabled people, set apart from those few individuals who have been 'normalised'.

● Commercial sponsorship of art and Disability Art

The acceptance of the medical model of disability has increased within society and arts practice with the arrival of biotechnology, which claims to provide the means of eradicating impairment. The dominance of global capitalism is evident in the proliferation of the same multinational companies throughout the world. The ethos of global capitalism has now even permeated into the arts; the most significant art commissions now available are through the likes of the Wellcome Trust and companies such as Gemini Gap whose operations are based on pseudo-scientific management principles. Funding opportunities within the public sector (the Arts Council of England (ACE), for example) now also align their commissioning agendas either directly or indirectly with those of commercial partners. This may be through direct partnership funding initiatives, such as ACE's with the Wellcome Trust. In sponsoring art and cultural events, companies are clearly trying to engage public support for their particular products, even if, like cigarettes, these are life-destroying rather than life-enhancing.

Unfortunately, as with most ideas which threaten the status quo, Disability Arts has been adopted by the mainstream not merely to neutralise its potential for socio-cultural disruption, but also to reinforce the original hegemony. It is quite logical that commercial partners would seek to validate their own commercial practices or products through arts commissioning, given the post-modern merging of art and advertising. Thus, more and more, biotechnology companies and other conglomerates, which have millions of pounds to spend on public relations, have used arts funding as a subtle way of gaining public support either for their practices or their products. It is no coincidence that, until now, cigarette companies, such as Gallagher, have used their wealth to fund a generation of modern artists. If they wish to enjoy the benefits of commercial sponsorship, then Disability Artists must appear to endorse the values of the companies which adopt them.

● State sponsorship of Disability Art

Since the initial period of hope for, and of, Disability Art, most regions linked to the English Regional Arts Board (RAB) funding system have developed and now run DAFs (Disability Arts Forums). The founding principles of DAFs are that they are run and controlled by disabled people combined with a belief in the social model of disability which frames and structures the work that they do. Yet this appearance of funding and support masks a more insidious reality. The proactive assertion of cultural assimilation is at the expense of actual cultural diversity. The centralisation of arts funding which took place in 2001 in the UK, with the abolition of the RABs and the creation of a regionalised Arts Council, will make little difference as almost all the same officers and cultural presumptions will remain.

Regional Arts Boards and the Arts Council of England, have used DAFs and Disability Art for a number of rather spurious reasons and Disability Artists and DAF organisers have often colluded rather than resisted. Other economically disadvantaged groups have also been 'bought off' with relatively small sums of money. For example, in the 2001 British General Election, the Labour Party promised to dedicate £150 million of National Lottery money to a number of especially poor and deprived towns and cities in the first few years of the new government. Whilst this sounds like a considerable sum of money, £150 million is less than the National Opera House alone received in Lottery funding for its rebuilding, never mind its running costs.

Superficially, it appears that Disability Art is being funded more generously than before and is being welcomed into the mainstream of contemporary art culture. Some argue that Disability Art is now so fully a part of our art culture that art historians, in order to re-evaluate the great art works and philosophies of the past, have started to appropriate it. However, Disability Artists still working with the memory of the original philosophy of Disability Art are more sceptical about both Disability Theory and, especially, about Disability Art. Such people argue that all 'equality' has meant in reality is that amongst the elite of the disabled community there is now a class of disabled people themselves exploiting other disabled people for their own career or financial benefit. Disabled people's culture has not been strengthened; what has resulted is the growth of the normalising hegemonies that oppress and deny the validity of disabled people *per se* which emanate from contemporary art cultures.

An example of such exploitation specific to regional Disability Arts was the creation of the West Midlands Disability Arts Forum (WMDAF) in 1996. The Regional Arts Board, West Midlands Arts, had previously funded an Art Link project. This organisation was a little like a DAF, but was not controlled and administered exclusively by disabled people although it did have a significant number of disabled board members and staff. The Regional Arts Board decided to withdraw Art Link's funding, which amounted to £70,000 per year in 1995. The process just described, which was carried out overnight and notified to Art Link by fax, put four full time staff out of work, two of whom were disabled people. Equally, it meant that nothing existed in relation to disabled people and art for the next year within that region. West Midlands Arts subsequently supported disabled people, including people from the Art Link organisation, to start up and secure National Lottery Charities Board funding of £40,000 per year for three years (1996–1999) for two staff, one full, one part time: WMDAF was founded. The reality, if looked at more broadly, was that West Midlands Arts (the RAB) had saved itself four years of funding commitments to the total of £280,000 in relation to disabled people and art and actually decreased disabled people's employment opportunities. It is important to note that West Midlands Arts actions can be seen as being in line with, and promoted by, a national Disability Arts agenda, set by the Arts Council for England.

The West Midlands Disability Arts Forum received almost no funding from the Regional Arts Board. In addition, WMDAF's work was to support and enable mainstream organisations within the region to attract and work with disabled people (mainly so that they could tick equal opportunities boxes and be seen to be working on audience development, not actually to make a difference). The conscious change was fundamentally about mainstreaming disabled artists, a practice that is very different to Disability Art and the work of Disability Artists. Mainstreaming is about reinforcing the existing structures, cultures and traditions of art practice; it is not about validating alternatives or even attempting to ameliorate the mainstream.

The Arts Council of England has been closely involved in the reconfiguration of the meaning of Disability Art. In 1995, a decision was made by ACE to close the Disability Arts Unit, known as the Access Unit. The number of staff working to support Disability Art was reduced to one part-timer. No matter how good that worker could be, it was a bitter blow to Disability Arts and, in retrospect, it sounded the death knell to Disability Art as a serious movement of any influence or significance. The situation was made worse by the fact that it happened just as arts funding received a 500 per cent increase, with the introduction of National Lottery Arts Funding through ACE. The National Lottery created a level of arts funding which, five years after the demise of the specialist Disability Arts team, was greater than the entire Arts Council budget in the previous 50 years. However, the lack of a specialist unit meant that there was no coherent strategy.

I would argue that, as a result of the submission of Disability Arts to ACE and its regional bodies, cultural diversity was replaced by the far more marginalising practice of cultural assimilation (though it was still labelled cultural diversity). Disability Art moved from being about wanting to change radically the nature of art and social culture, to being used by many disabled people (at the insistence of funding remits) to say: 'I want to be in your gang' or 'I want to be valued by traditional art culture and history'. Disability Art took a direction that soon defeated all of its own original aims and intentions, a direction that has meant that the majority of disabled people, and Disability Artists, are in a worse situation than they had been in before.

As a result of the additional funding described above, many disabled people from the Disability Arts movement moved into the institutions which had for so long excluded them, taking up well-paid jobs linked to equal opportunities, issues of access, employment and training disabled people in the traditions of the culture that had previously excluded them. We all took our share of the thirty pieces of silver and will have to continue doing so to maintain our status, lifestyle and apparent high degree of normalised habitus and cultural capital. Current practices and processes actually do little for the majority of disabled people, but create a situation where the more normalised disabled people will not be as excluded as they were before, at least superficially. The acceptance of a small number of Disabled Artists is in line with the parading of the assimilated disabled – people such as paralympians, ex- or current models, the sons and daughters of the rich and educated and other televisual tokens. Such individuals never complain of being disabled but keenly discuss impairment, thereby ensuring the individualisation of the social in order to further mystify the real socio-political issues of disablement (Oliver 1990). These supposed role models are representatives of a normalised education, consumer, ambition, class and/or morality or as the normalised acceptable face of difference. In fact, they negate the entire notion of difference in the process of reinforcing the hegemony, the values, the 'hope', of conformity and normality, often in association with consumerist fantasies and idealisations of youth and wealth.

This is not to question the sincerity of the motivations of any individual or group. However, given the nature of a culture rooted in the hegemony of normality, it is impossible not to collude in it if one is to achieve any degree of success. Consequently, collusion and 'forgetfulness' (betrayal) was unavoidable given the threat that Disability Art posed to mainstream society and culture. Success, even survival, meant adaptation and a very long sip at the river of Lethe, where, as Plato wrote, forgetfulness was the only nourishment possible for future life. Most disabled people who are successful have played the game and have been rewarded for their complicity as a consequence. A culturally normalised habitus, open to a few disabled people, is what has been developed amongst some disabled artists and administrators. Disability Art has been well and truly displaced in the name of a greater hegemonic good of normality.

Despite the absorption of a small number of Disability Artists, the working lives of the majority have become increasingly fragmented. Individual Disability Artists wander from one small commission to another, filling the void with equal opportunities training or audience development initiatives to legitimate the big bucks, usually from the National Lottery, that go to the mainstream organisations. In addition DAFs, or their kind, provide palliative project work for local authorities to relieve the boredom of day centre attendees, or empire-build with a view to job security by clinging like barnacles to key strategic organisations and venues within their own and neighbouring regions. All the while national Disability Arts organisations hold conferences and seminars for mainstream organisations, begging to be let in to the club of the big boys, whilst they search for funding and the survival of their organisation.

The domestication of Disability Art and Disability Artists

Highly significant in relation to the commodification of art is the way in which 'high' art has become the preserve of elite groups, reflecting their cultural habitus. The idea of habitus was developed by Bourdieu (1993) to describe the norms, values, practices and ideologies of a particular social class group which are so much part of its way of life as to be accepted unconsciously and uncritically. Appreciation of art is part of bourgeois habitus and art therefore attracts the support of elite groups. In relation to high art, the 'general public' is fundamentally an irrelevance. Thus, acceptance within the culture of mainstream art means taking on the habitus of that culture to pass or succeed within it.

Initially, Disability Art challenged the particular tradition that defines what is and is not art. Disability Art did not fit the codes of the past or the present art capital or art habitus of the mainstream, a fact which meant that it was, at least initially, culturally incomprehensible. Establishment art culture, when faced with a new culture rejecting the traditional values of the art world, was understandably shocked, bewildered and a little resistant. Disability Art, in attempting to create a culture of disabled people revelling in opposition to the dominant hegemonies of normality oppression, went further than being a mere rupture; it undermined the core values and revealed the processes of mainstream cultural construction.

In order to neutralise this threat, attempts have been made by the guardians of traditional art to assimilate Disability Art into the established tradition. Thus, disabled artists are now supported more than ever in getting into art schools to train in the traditions of art creation, under-standing, history and appreciation. The aim is to absorb them into the mainstream tradition. Disability Art, on the other hand, is not taught at all except in its distorted form linked to Community Arts. The way of seeing (to quote John Berger's famous phrase) has not changed at all; all that has happened is that some disabled people are now allowed to experience the privileges of the few in the appreciation of what is the current notion of art.

As a result of existing art hierarchies, Disability Art events, exhibi-tions and performances are invariably marginalised as art *per se* or held purely as education-based events. There is almost never a single artist exhibition of a Disability Artist, for example, there are only ever collective exhibitions. The only disabled artists who get such showcases completely deny any relevance to Disability Art or even the notion of a social model of disability. Instead, such artists are fêted as inspirational role models despite being, for example, 'severely crippled with arthritis' or having overcome so 'heroically' the onset of paralysis.

According to Bourdieu, for the establishment, who control art cap-ital, art is not art if it is mere communication or education. Disability Art has been distorted to become a tool simply to address issues such as 'disability' access, training and audience development. This has under-mined the capacity of Disability Art to develop a serious philosophy and to contribute to the culture of disabled people. The art establishment(s) take any Disability Equality Training (DET) offered, which is almost compulsory in any Lottery Arts funding application. This means that Disability Art is seen as nothing other than either education or a means of communicating an awareness of a social issue. The response of Dis-ability Artists to these pressures has varied. Some have made work which is increasingly simplistic or shallow in content, and work that is overtly political or propagandist in relation to the social model of disability. A large number of Disabled Artists specialise in Disability Equality Training linked to an exhibition or event. Whilst such work may have some value, it is something which black, women or gay artists ceased to do years ago and which 'normal' artists have never done. Unfortunately this reduces art to mere communication or education in content, meaning and theory. It means that Disabled Artists are not allowed to be 'difficult', but, as Bourdieu has noted 'difficulty' is what is valued within bourgeois art.

As noted above, a small number of Disabled Artists, who can operate within a traditional art habitus, are allowed to participate in the world of traditional art and their existence increases the sense of satisfaction the tradition has with itself. By allowing the 'right type' of artist entry to the tradition, the tradition reassures itself that it is acces-sible to those of real worth. In order to be admitted to this world, one must demonstrate that one has mastered art classifications and is able to incorporate them into one's own work. Such knowledge is the language that allows artists to 'speak' directly to an art establishment figure and/or venue without ever having to speak a word. It is a secret language that permits exclusion of those who challenge or seek to access it. The establishment processes that have been set up, whereby individuals or bodies from the art establishment sit in judgement on funding applications from artists or organisations, merely serve to reinforce the negation of Disability Art and the apparent mainstream success of 'artists with disabilities'.

Disability Artists are, in reality, in a no-win situation. Often they have no education or training in the traditions of the art habitus and, if they do, they are only allowed within the inner sanctum of art production if they reinforce those values. Thus, the issue is not the morality of any individual artist but the nature of the culture of art and society itself (the original point of Disability Art). Those individual 'artists with disabilities' who have been allowed to practise within the traditions of art culture will, and often do, take vociferous exception to Disability Art and Disability Artists, on the basis of their own fragile sense of themselves masquerading as 'normal' in a non-normal body. Consequently, much of their work is often about their own bodies or, in extreme opposition, completely avoids the body as an issue and takes flight in obsessions with facile beauty and normality. Criticisms of the marginalisation of Disability Art are met by such artists with accusations of envy, jealousy and bitterness.

Bourdieu's (1993) observations on the creation and use of cultural capital are particularly relevant to Disability Art. He urges us:

> To remember that culture is not what one is but what one has, or rather, what one becomes; to remember the social conditions which render possible aesthetic experience of those beings – art lovers or 'people of taste' – for whom it is possible; to remember that the work of art is given only to those who have received the means to acquire the means to appropriate it and who could seek to possess it if they did not already possess it, in and through the possession of means of possession as an actual possibility of effecting the taking of possession; to remember, finally, that only a few have the real possibility of benefiting from the theoretical possibility, generously offered to all, of taking advantage of the works exhibited in museums – all this is to bring to light the hidden force of the effects of the majority of culture's social uses.   (Bourdieu 1993, p. 234)

Conclusion

Finally, I believe that the Disability Art movement has been lost except in the activity of a few Disabled Artists who work at the margins not just of art culture, but of culture more widely. The original aims of Disability Art have been forgotten, as Disability Artists have taken so many sips from the river Lethe (increasingly irrigated across the UK by National Lottery funding!). The core aim of Disability Arts was never to be part of a hegemony of normality (mainstream art culture) to be redefining what normality (primarily within art culture) is: a fantasy. All that is left now is the hope that one day there may be a culture of disabled people. If such a culture does develop, it will not emerge from Disability Art as it is now configured within mainstream arts culture, but from the practices and theories of disabled people.

Disability Art was an art practice with a theoretical basis that was about revealing the 'hidden force of the effects of the majority culture's social uses', not just in relation to disabled people but all people. Too many of us have forgotten the theoretical basis of the Disability Art movement, and the success of a few Disability Artists has been at the expense of the many. As a result, Disability Art and Disability Artists have become, largely through no fault of their own, a tool of the 'hidden forces' used against disabled people to legitimise their (our) continued mass exclusion from not just art culture but culture more widely.

Acknowledgement

I would like to thank the artist Ann Whitehurst for her assistance in the formulation of this chapter through general discussions, in making comments specific to Disability Art and in raising questions about the content and wider implications of the argument developed here. Without her assistance, I would have not been able to write this chapter.

References

Bourdieu, P. (1993) 'A Sociology Theory of Art Perception' in Bourdieu, P. (ed.) *The Field of Cultural Production*, Polity Press, Cambridge.

Bowler, A. (1994) 'Methodological dilemmas in the sociology of art' in Crane, D. (ed.) *The Sociology of Culture*, Blackwell, Oxford.

Campbell, J. and Oliver, M. (1996) *Disability Politics*, Routledge, London.

Crane, D. (ed.) (1994) *The Sociology of Culture*, Blackwell, Oxford.

Crow, E. (1995) *Disability Arts: The Business*, National Disability Arts Forum (NDAF), Newcastle-upon-Tyne.

Morrison, E. (1990) *Dail Magazine: Anthology The First Five Years*, LDAF, London.

Oliver, M. (1990) *The Politics of Disablement*, Macmillan, Basingstoke.

CHAPTER 9

Mainstreaming disability on Radio 4

Brian Sweeney and Sheila Riddell

Introduction

In 1997, the controller of Radio 4, James Boyle, announced a decision to reorganise the coverage of disability issues of Radio 4 as part of a wider rescheduling initiative which took place the following year. The programme *Does He Take Sugar? (DHTS?)*, which had covered disability issues since the 1970s, was axed. The team which had produced *DHTS?* was redeployed to *You and Yours (Y&Y)*, a consumer affairs programme. Before rescheduling, *Y&Y* had a 35-minute slot; this was increased to fifty minutes (12.05–12.55 p.m. daily). Peter White, a blind broadcaster, was appointed to the post of disability correspondent, with a remit to ensure that disability featured in programmes right across the network. Whilst mainstreaming disability was the order of the day, *In Touch*, a programme dealing with issues relevant to blind and visually impaired people, was retained.

The rescheduling initiative promoted much discussion about the treatment of disability on the radio and in the media more generally. It raised questions about the power of the media to influence people's understanding of disability, the arguments for and against mainstreaming versus specialist approaches to disability in culture and social policy and the significance of a consumerist approach to disability issues. These questions became the central focus of Brian Sweeney's PhD research, which began in 1998 shortly after the decision to reschedule. In considering the treatment of disability on Radio 4, the research focused on three key areas·

▓   What production decisions and values influenced changes in the treatment of disability on Radio 4?

▓   What messages about disability were embedded in the content of programmes before and after rescheduling?

▓   How did audiences of disabled and non-disabled people make sense of the programmes before and after rescheduling with regard to the treatment of disability?

This focus on production, content and reception informed a rolling programme of work in the Glasgow Media Research Group, where Jenny Kitzinger, one of Brian's supervisors, was working at the start of the research. One theme of the Glasgow Media Research Group's work has been the power of the media to influence popular opinion through the propagation of negative stereotypes of disabled people in relation, for example, to mental illness (Philo 1996) and HIV/Aids (Kitzinger 1993). The work reported here thus draws on both methodological and substantive concerns within media studies.

This chapter addresses production and content matters, considering the intentions of the controller and programme producers with regard to the treatment of disability pre- and post-rescheduling and the ways in which these intentions were reflected in programme content and tone. Six key informant interviews were conducted with central players in order to explore production issues. Content analysis explored the treatment of disability issues pre- and post- rescheduling with a particular focus on *Does He Take Sugar?* and *You and Yours*. Other programmes post-rescheduling were also examined, such as *No Triumph No Tragedy*, but these are not discussed in this chaper. The analysis presented here is based on ten editions of *DHTS?* recorded during 1997 and 1998. In addition, a sample of *Y&Y* programmes for September 1998, 1999 and 2000 were recorded and analysed. Tables were produced which summarised and quantified basic features of the programmes, for instance the length of particular items, the nature of the impairment which they considered and the broad topic of each item. Programme synopses were also produced, and these were analysed qualitatively in order to understand the discourses of disability which they reflected. Of particular interest here was the extent to which there had been a shift in the conceptualisation of disability from a collective political issue in *DHTS?* to an individualised consumer issue in *Y&Y*. Audience response to the changes were investigated through a series of focus groups.

In this chapter, we first consider some key conceptual issues. Subsequently, we present data from key informant interviews and programme content analysis to explore shifts in disability discourses pre- and post-rescheduling.

Media, power and disability

Within media and cultural studies, there are long-standing debates about the power of the mass media to influence the way in which people think and behave. These debates have been particularly heated in relation to sensitive issues such as the extent to which the portrayal of violence on television and in films encourages people to emulate such behaviour in real life. For example, it was widely reported in coverage of the James Bulger case that Venables and Thompson, the child murderers, had watched a video (*Chuckie*) in which a toy comes to life and carries out acts of extreme violence. Eldridge, Kitzinger and Williams (1997) note the widespread belief that modern mass communication media exert a total and all-embracing power. This fear of the media is, however, a recurrent anxiety rather than a uniquely modern phenomenon:

> . . . The history of mass communication shows the emergence of every new medium of mass communication or popular amusement has been accompanied by great claims about the power of the medium to change the behaviour of men, women and children as well as the values and mores of society.   (Eldridge, Kitzinger and Williams 1997, p. 10)

Researchers in media and cultural studies have sometimes argued the converse case, that audiences are active, not passive, and have considerable power to subvert or resist the messages transmitted by the media. Kitzinger (1999) suggests that:

> Concepts such as 'polysemy', 'resistance' and 'the active audience' are often used to by-pass or even negate enquiry into the effects of cinema, press or televisual representations. Our work [that of the Glasgow Media Research Group] shows that the complex processes of reception and consumption *mediate*, but do not necessarily *undermine*, media power. Acknowledging that audiences can be 'active' does not mean that the media are ineffectual. Recognising the role of interpretation does not invalidate the concept of influence.   (Kitzinger 1999, p. 4)

This research is based on the assumption that producers of radio programmes have intentions *vis à vis* content and tone, although these are not always clear and rational but may be poorly articulated or confused. It also assumes that production values and intentions are reflected in programme content, so that messages are transmitted to listeners, although these messages may also be complex and conflicting rather than clear and consistent. Finally, an assumption is made that audiences do not simply read and absorb messages, but interpret them in the light of their existing social and individual schemata, rejecting some, reorganising others and readily accepting those which reinforce their existing world-view. For these reasons, it is important to understand the way in which the media construe disability, because this will have an important effect on the creation of wider cultural understandings.

Inclusion, exclusion and mainstreaming

The debate about whether disability should be dealt with in a separate specialist slot or incorporated into general programmes brings us to the heart of debates about the politics of representation which have been tackled by feminists such as Phillips (1997; 1999) and Young (1990). Traditional class politics were based on the idea that society was made up of groups with discrete and conflicting economic interests. More recently, there has been a recognition of the complexity, multiplicity and transience of individual identity or identities (see, for example, Watson, Ferguson and Meekosha, this volume). Such questions had particular salience for the founding fathers of the disability movement. Writers like Oliver (1990) and Barnes (1991) adopted Marxist arguments to maintain that disabled people should be seen as a group experiencing particular forms of economic oppression which led to their social and political marginalisation. These writers maintained that impairment should be sidelined as a concept; it was not useful to think about the particular experiences of people with learning difficulties, mental health problems or sensory impairments because this undermined the unity of the disabled people's movement and the social model of disability which formed its basis. More recently, a range of writers (Shakespeare and Watson 2001; Thomas 1999) have suggested the need to recognise the complexity of disabled people's experiences and identities, even if this may have a political cost.

As we will see in the following section, one of the reasons for the demise of *DHTS?* was that it was seen as promoting an overly simplified view of disability, although building a sense of shared identity was also seen as one of its strengths. Similarly, attempts to 'normalise' disability by including it as part of mainstream features in Y&Y may be seen as positive, in terms of transmitting the message that 'disabled people are just the same as everyone else', or it may serve to undermine the shared political and cultural identity which the disability movement has sought to nurture. In addition, attempts to emphasise universality may obscure differences in group experiences which need to be recognised so that injustice may be redressed. The positions adopted by the Controller of Radio 4 and members of the production team are discussed below.

Rights, citizenship and consumerism

The decision to move disability issues from *DHTS?* to *Y&Y* was seen as a shift towards consumerism and it is therefore important to sketch the evolution of this approach. Marshall (1950) argued that citizenship entailed access to civil, political and social rights and obligations. Whereas traditional notions of citizenship had emphasised civil and political rights, Marshall considered that these rights had effectively been won. However, he suggested, individuals needed access to employment, education and a decent standard of living in order to enjoy full social participation. These ideas have been highly influential in shaping the post-war welfare agenda (see, for example, the Borrie Report 1994). As the interest of policy-makers in citizenship increased, it became evident that a more subtle and nuanced understanding of the concept was required to avoid universalising the experience of a small and privileged group of white, middle-class men. Lister (1997), for example, considered the ways in which the concept needed to be expanded to embrace the experiences of a range of women.

During the 1990s, a new conception of citizenship emerged, emphasising the citizen as consumer. The Citizen's Charter, the 'big idea' of John Major's Conservative administration, cast the consumer as an individual, rather than a member of a group, challenging bureaucracies to deliver adequate services and seeking means of complaint and redress. The notion of citizen as consumer fitted neatly with the promotion of the market as the final social arbiter, an idea which was championed by right-wing economists such as von Hayek and Friedman and which found favour with Conservative politicians on both sides of the Atlantic (Deakin 1994). Throughout the 1990s there was a growing emphasis on access to information and choice in both the public and the private sector, alongside access to means of complaint and redress. According to market theorists, the good society arises as a result of individuals choosing services which best meet their needs. If the free flow of money is permitted, then 'good' services (i.e. those which are chosen by the greatest number of individuals) will flourish and 'bad' services will disappear. There are of course a number of flaws in this argument which have frequently been noted, such as the fact that there is no guarantee that aggregated individual choices will produce good collective outcomes. For example, the decision by most people to drive cars produces negative consequences for society as a whole in terms of road deaths, pollution, noise and environmental destruction. In addition, citizens who do not use particular services, such as schools, may well have an interest in determining what form these should take because education provides benefits for the whole of society, not just those whose children are currently in school. In general, consumerism emphasises individual actions and lifestyles and de-emphasises collective identity and action. Thus the decision to shift coverage of disability into a programme with an explicit consumerist orientation implies a particular conception of disabled people as individuals rather than as members of a political movement with common interests.

Having explained the background to the research and outlined some of its key conceptual concerns, we now explore some of the insights gleaned from key informant interviews concerning struggles over production decisions.

Production issues

Three central perspectives are considered here, those of the Controller of Radio 4, the *DHTS?* production team and the production team of *Y&Y*.

The Controller's perspective

The Controller of Radio 4 explained that his decision to cut *DHTS?* was because it acted as a 'ghetto', preventing other programmes from tackling disability issues. Considering whether *DHTS?* was a useful programme, he concluded that:

> It was simply not true that the programme had any special cachet for disabled people. And the second thing was that it was actually denying disability within the mainstream.

Because 'we had simultaneously decided that consumerism itself was going to be an extremely important part of the schedule', it was decided to relocate *DHTS?* within the *Y&Y* slot and reframe disability as a consumerist issue. Retaining a specialist slot for disabled people was, according to the Controller, locating them as different in a stigmatising way:

> ...we were making a programme for...people who wanted to define themselves as disabled. And for a public who wanted to define them as disabled. And in that respect...they were 'off the norm' because they weren't able-bodied. They were disabled. And, therefore, everything that was in that programme was going to be about that particular function of their lives...We wanted to move it into the middle and say to people 'Look, these people actually do not respond to radio and television like that. Because they are not *these people* – they are the same as the rest of us...' So, I wanted to move it into the consumer model so that it was part of an array of choices for the general public, some of whom are disabled.

Implicit in the Controller's comments is the view that it is not legitimate for disabled people to define themselves as different from other people and an assumption that adopting a disabled identity is automatically stigmatising rather than positive. This assumption is also evident when he describes *DHTS?* as adopting a medical model by seeing disabled people as different from others. He counterpoises the medical model of *DHTS?* with the social model of *Y&Y*, which he defines as synonymous with the consumer model. This represents an interesting slippage in terminology, since *DHTS?* frequently featured proponents of the social model such as Professor Mike Oliver. In addition the very title of the programme, *Does He Take Sugar?* implicitly mocks the medical model of disability which assumes that individuals can be defined, negatively, by their deficit. However, this confusion is consistent with the Controller's assumption that adopting the identity of a disabled person is essentially a negative act.

The Controller believed that the mainstreaming of disability had been successful and there was much more coverage of disability issues right across the network. He also felt that the dispersal of the team of disabled people who had been responsible for the production of *DHTS?* was positive:

> Take (name of individual): he moved over to Westminster reporting. Having frankly been stuck in a programme about the disabled for a long time... I think that was part of just *encouraging* people to see their careers more broadly. Because you're disabled, because you're blind or in a chair, you don't need to be doing disabled programmes.

The central mistake the Controller acknowledged was retaining *In Touch* as a specialist slot:

> I have to say that in some respects we got *In Touch* wrong. Because I believed it when I was told that there's a special relationship between radio and the blind... and it came out about a couple of years after we made the changes that there wasn't any special relationship and there was no greater incidence of listening to *In Touch* by blind people than anyone else. I should have known that, but I allowed my heart to rule my head.

From the Controller's perspective, the idea of mainstreaming disability was incompatible with retaining specialist programmes:

> You can't have one unit saying 'It's a special thing for a small group of people – we'll put our resources in there' – and others saying, 'No, it's a general story'.

The *DHTS?* team perspective

A very different view was presented by members of the *DHTS?* production team. One key informant noted a number of problems with the idea and implementation of mainstreaming, but also some positive outcomes. He took issue with the idea that only a small group of disabled people listened to *DHTS?* and *In Touch*. RAJAR listening data indicated that audiences for *DHTS?* (9.30 p.m. – 10.00 p.m. on Thursdays) were higher than was normal for that time slot on other evenings of the week. A significant proportion of listeners were 'eavesdroppers', that is, people who were not necessarily already knowledgeable about disability, and perhaps started listening by chance, but were subsequently intrigued by the subject matter and became regular listeners. Because *DHTS?* and *In Touch* were aimed at a core audience who were already well informed about disability issues and politics, they could go into considerable depth, educating the 'eavesdroppers' *en route*. Mainstream programmes like *Y&Y*, by way of contrast, were not able to assume prior knowledge of disability issues and were therefore able to tackle particular topics in a relatively superficial way. The advantages of assuming prior knowledge were explained thus:

> I think the intelligent listener actually gains, in a way, from not having been hit over the head with the concepts but being made to understand them as you go along. In a way that you do when you eavesdrop. When you eavesdrop, you put it together . . . You say, 'What's this about? What's that about?' And I think there's a sense of that with disability programmes.   (Member of *DHTS?* production team)

It was felt by members of the *DHTS?* production team that a major reason for cutting disability programmes was that :

> . . . they could be a prisoner of the interest groups. They could be a prisoner of the charities, they could be a prisoner of the more radical disability organisations etc . . . Unpoliticised disabled people might not feel as included as . . . more committed, more politically placed groups.
>   (Member of *DHTS?* production team)

In fact, it was stated, there was probably more of a danger that this would take place within the context of mainstreaming:

> . . . where there's perhaps less specialist knowledge, [programmes are] more likely to be captivated or captured by more organised groups with good PR, than a specialist programme which knows its area and its subjects well and knows who's who and who's peddling what . . . I think the view was that groups could have a free hit on disability programmes and he wanted to stop that.   (Member of *DHTS?* production team)

Members of the DHTS? production team felt that, since rescheduling, *Y&Y* had 'honoured its remit' to be the principal place where disability issues are addressed in the schedule within the programme's consumer/lifestyle format. Indeed, *Y&Y* often included, per week, more items about disability than had been covered in *DHTS?*. However, as noted earlier, items were shortened and were dealt with in less depth. In addition, disabled people no longer knew when disability issues would be covered on the network. What was sacrificed was:

> ...the certainty of knowing where the coverage actually is. Because we're talking about being in a programme which goes out for an hour every day and, you know, if you gave it a slot, then you might as well just have kept *Sugar*. So they haven't done that. But in terms of identifying where it is, that would be quite difficult for an audience which says, 'I can't listen to a programme for an hour every day, so when will I know when a disability issue will crop up?'

In this way, the sense of a community of disabled people, with a shared identity, had been disrupted by the removal of *DHTS?*.

A further blow to the development of the political movement of disabled people arose as a result of the dispersal of the production team. *DHTS?* had its roots in the 1970s when the disability movement was growing as a civil rights movement alongside the women's movement and other new social movements. Issues of representation were at the centre of the disability movement's thinking, sparking major debates about who had the right to reflect the views of disabled people in research (Barnes 1996; Shakespeare 1996; Riddell *et al.*, 1998) and in culture (Barnes 1992; Shakespeare 1994). *DHTS?* nurtured a production team, which, by the late 1990s, was made up entirely of disabled people connected to the disability movement. This enabled a certain tone to be adopted which assumed a shared base of knowledge and understanding, or 'standpoint', between the programme presenters and listeners. A member of the *DHTS?* production team explained that this shared identity allowed a particular tone to be adopted:

> You can take a tone... which actually uses the word 'we' quite a lot. So, if a presenter has a disability that's a natural, not a pretentious thing to do, and you actually talk from the point of view of inclusiveness. As opposed to 'these rather odd people and these are the problems they have'. Now I'm not suggesting that *Y&Y* does that, or any other programme does that, but it's subtle and it's very hard not to be implied. Whereas programmes like *Sugar* were able to say: 'we're able to talk to

> people from the inside'. And I don't think we've got to the point
> (in the political development of the disability movement) where that
> isn't necessary.

Members of the *DHTS?* production team believed that it should be possible to have disability 'woven throughout the schedule', whilst preserving specialist slots aimed at people who need depth of coverage because 'disability is a major part of their lives'. An analogy was drawn between the coverage of motoring issues on the media. There is room for a programme like *Top Gear*, aimed at people who are 'bonkers about cars', but also for a different type of coverage in other programmes aimed at people for whom cars are not the major source of interest.

Whereas the Controller believed that treatment of disability issues was significantly better post-rescheduling, members of the *DHTS?* production team had reservations. It was believed that the project of mainstreaming disability across the network had been only partially successful. Some producers were very keen to cover disability issues, whilst some paid lip-service to the idea but did little in reality. It was felt that some excellent programmes had been commissioned post-rescheduling (*No Triumph, No Tragedy* was seen as a prime example of a programme which combined both personal and political insights into understandings of disability). However, there was a danger that, without the training ground provided by *DHTS?* for young disabled broadcasters to develop their skills, such programmes might not be produced in the future.

Finally, *DHTS?* production team members questioned the process by which the decision to reschedule had been made. The Controller made this decision in isolation and without consulting key groups. Research was cited in support of the decision to mainstream disability, but *DHTS?* members did not think that the research actually supported the decisions which were taken. A monitoring group, with representation from a range of voluntary organisations, but not groups of disabled people, was set up and had a number of meetings following the reorganisation. However, the remit of the group was unclear and it was disbanded without producing a report.

The *Y&Y* production team's perspective

An interview with a key member of the *Y&Y* production team elicited insights into the type of debates which had taken place concerning the incorporation of disability issues into the programme. Initially, it was felt that disability issues should be dealt with on a particular day so that listeners would know where they were located, but this idea was soon abandoned. There were some early difficulties in amalgamating the *DHTS?* and *Y&Y* teams:

When the *DHTS?* team started working with us, there was a suspicion that disability stories wouldn't get on air. When and if they did get on air, it was also felt that a disabled reporter wouldn't be doing the lead story.

Such fears, she felt, were largely unfounded and the amalgamation of the two teams was relatively unproblematic. She believed that *Y&Y* had broadened the scope of its coverage and now dealt with a range of issues including 'lifestyle, leisure, disabilities, environmental, transport, travel . . .'. She preferred to think of it as a magazine rather than a purely consumer programme (although clearly the list of topics covered suggests a focus on the individual consumer rather than a broader social or political stance). There was, a difficulty, she acknowledged, in dealing with what she termed 'documentary' issues or significant political developments such as the establishment of the Disability Rights Commission:

That's the sort of thing where I would say you could actually have a landmark event. And it's difficult to put a landmark event within a magazine programme.

Finally, coverage of disability issues was constrained by reactions of the general public and of the *Y&Y* team:

I did get a letter a few weeks ago saying, 'You're always moaning on about people with disabilities. Why are you bothering with them'. You will get that. The other thing I've had from members of the team is 'Oh, that's going to be a bit worthy isn't it?'.

To summarise, key informant interviews revealed very clearly the positions of the Controller and the *DHTS?* team. Whereas the former saw specialist disability programmes as inherently ghettoising and stigmatising, members of the *DHTS?* team felt that the programme had played a key role in building disabled people's collective consciousness. Comments by a member of the *Y&Y* production team illustrated the constraints in dealing seriously with political issues on a consumerist programme. Speaking about oppression was, in her view, likely to be seen as 'moaning' or 'worthy'.

Content

As indicated above, a systematic analysis was undertaken of the length, substance and tone of items on *DHTS?* and *Y&Y* over a specified period of time. On average, it appeared that individual items on disability were given more time on *DHTS?* than *Y&Y*. The average airtime on the former programme was nine minutes and three seconds, whereas on the latter it was seven minutes and twelve seconds. On average, *DHTS?* devoted slightly more time per week to disability issues than *Y&Y* (thirty minutes as opposed to twenty-eight minutes). However, there was great variation in the amount of time devoted to disability issues in *Y&Y* each week, and on some days there was no coverage at all.

Because of its specialist nature, *DHTS?* was able to devote a considerable length of time to particular items if they were judged to merit in-depth treatment. For example, a report of a Direct Action Network demonstration in Bristol against restricted access to public transport was given twenty-eight minutes. This type of item would be unlikely to be covered in *Y&Y* because, whilst transport lends itself to being addressed as a consumer issue, discussion of political tactics is not readily tackled in a lifestyle format. A transport item in *Y&Y* might typically consist of a short item dealing with the problems encountered by a disabled person in persuading an airline to carry their wheelchair without an additional charge.

Whereas there was some similarity in the type of items covered, the nature of their treatment varied. This point may be illustrated by contrasting the coverage of two items dealing with 'cures' for impairments. An item on *DHTS?* on 11 September 1997, lasting 13 minutes, dealt with the efficacy of spinal implant surgery for people who had become wheelchair users as a result of an injury. Frederick Dove, who presented the item, posed some questions in his introduction:

> The public is, perhaps understandably, fascinated by the possibility
> of people who've been paralysed being made to walk again. The
> unsuccessful attempts of PC Olds to dispense with his wheelchair, and
> the declared intent of Christopher 'Superman' Reeves to walk again,
> have fuelled the idea that a miracle cure is just around the corner.
> Even quite modest claims, such as the latest results of a spinal implant
> programme undertaken by London's University College and published
> in *The Lancet*, have given rise to a batch of highly optimistic headlines.
> But what do such projects really involve and what are the realistic aims
> of people with spinal injuries? And do irresponsible publicity and the
> expectations of society put unfair pressure on those who are paralysed
> to believe they must walk at any cost?

The item went on to explore technical aspects of the treatment and criticisms of the biomedical approach by a disabled person who argued that they reinforced unhelpful views of being able to walk as essential to enjoying a high quality of life. The views of a disabled woman, Julie Hill, who had undergone spinal implant surgery, were also presented. Julie insisted that she was aware of the treatment's limitations and her reasons for wanting the treatment had nothing to do with image or false hopes:

> I had absolutely no thoughts of miracle cures at all. I knew this was
> going to be hard work. I knew it was research and, as I said, if we could
> get to a point where I could stand, using this, then brilliant! ... I never
> felt it was the be-all and end-all. I've had a very, very good life in a
> wheelchair.

Subsequently, the programme went on to discuss the politics and economics of the search to 'cure' people of impairments, and the balance that should be struck between investing in expensive medical research and transforming society to accommodate people with diverse needs. Overall, the programme was clearly located within a social model of disability discourse, but succeeded in interrogating alternative positions in a way which did not simply dismiss them as misguided or wrong. Its presenter, Frederick Dove, and reporter, Peter White, would both be recognised as prominent disabled broadcasters with a thorough understanding of disability politics, and this shared but unstated understanding informed the tone of the programme.

A similar programme on *Y&Y* on 16 September 1998 included an item which dealt with a week-long campaign mounted by the Association for Spina Bifida and Hydrocephalus (ASBAH). The campaign sought to raise awareness of and change attitudes towards people with spina bifida, but was sponsored by a pharmaceutical company which manufactured and marketed folic acid supplements for pregnant women, with a view to reducing the chances of a baby being born with spina bifida. Following the introduction, there was a discussion between Tony Britten, ASBAH's communications manager, and Paul Darke, introduced as 'a disability campaigner who has spina bifida'.

Liz Barclay, a non-disabled presenter, asked Paul Darke what he found problematic about the message ASBAH was trying to promote. Darke replied that ASBAH should be focusing on promoting the interests of people with spina bifida and that responsibility for the promotion of folic acid should lie with the Department of Health. By appearing to argue that people with spina bifida should not be born, ASBAH was contributing to a negative image. In addition, ASBAH was an organisation for people with spina bifida but run by and large by non-disabled people, which again promoted a negative stereotype. In contrast to Darke's complex argument, Tony Britten simply stated that ASBAH's role was:

> To help ensure disabled people have equal opportunities to lead successful and fulfilled lives. That's about people who are alive . . . Not supporting a policy to stop them being born.

The item lasted only four minutes, and the listener was likely to be left confused by Darke's argument because there was insufficient time for it to be fully developed and contextualised. Britten's much more simple argument, by way of contrast, appeared to be far more in keeping with programmes 'soundbite' approach. The listener who was unfamiliar with the struggles of disabled people against eugenics was unlikely to understand why Darke should be making these points, instead of welcoming a week's campaign to raise awareness of a particular condition. The fact that the programme was presented by a non-disabled woman was also likely to promote a view that disabled people were 'a rather odd group' (see above). This contrasted with the fact that Dove and White, as disabled presenters of *DHTS?*, were able to speak with the authority of experience.

Conclusion

The decision to mainstream disability issues on Radio 4 raises many interesting issues about the role of the media in contributing to cultural representations of disabled people. *DHTS?* was ostensibly cut because it was not attracting a large enough audience, but the Controller explained that there were also important political and ideological reasons for its demise. His view was that a programme reflecting a political perspective on disability was outmoded and was ultimately stigmatising of disabled people by underlining their difference from others. A similar argument could of course have been made in relation to *Woman's Hour*, but in this case the political outcry at its removal might have been too great. The argument of members of the *DHTS?* production team, that it should be possible to deal with disability issues in both specialist and mainstream contexts, was dismissed. Their argument, that the treatment of disability issues on *Y&Y* would lack political bite, appears to have been borne out by the content analysis of the two programmes conducted as part of this research. If disability issues are located within a consumer programme, then it is likely that the focus will be on individual lifestyle preferences and the broader social, political and economic forces which shape individual choices will be ignored. The *DHTS?* production team maintained that the disability movement has drawn strength from recognising these structural factors, and programmes like *DHTS?* have been instrumental in developing such understandings. There is a danger that the removal of such programmes may contribute to the depoliticisation of the disabled people's movement.

Finally, it is interesting to consider why the demise of *DHTS?* was accepted with relative equanimity by disabled people. If, as its production team claimed, the programme sought to develop a shared sense of what it means to be a disabled person, then the removal of the programme might have been seen as an attack on disabled people's culture and a vigorous, rather than muted response might have been expected. Barnes and Mercer (2001) have noted that:

> ... the generation of a separate cultural identity has divided disabled people. While some groups, such as deaf people, have long regarded themselves as having a distinctive culture, most disabled people have been less enthusiastic. (Barnes and Mercer 2001, p. 525)

Since many disabled people have experienced segregation in negative terms, then deliberately seeking out a separate cultural identity may seem perverse. Whilst *DHTS?* sought to develop a positive image of disabled people to counteract pervasive negative social attitudes, it is possible that many disabled people did not share this vision, regarding the existence of a separate programme for disabled people as supporting, rather than challenging, negative stereotypes.

References

Barnes, C. (1991) *Disabled People in Britain and Discrimination*, Hurst & Co, London.

Barnes, C. (1992) *Disabling Imagery and the Media: An Exploration of Media Representations of Disabled People*, British Council of Organisations of Disabled People, Belper.

Barnes, C. (1996) 'Disability and the myth of the independent researcher' in *Disability and Society*, 2(1), pp. 107–111.

Barnes, C. and Mercer, G. (2001) 'Disability culture: Assimilation or inclusion?' in Albrecht, G.L., Seelman, K.D. and Bury, M. (eds) *Handbook of Disability Studies*, Sage, London.

Deakin, N. (1994) *The Politics of Welfare: Continuity and Change*, Harvester Wheatsheaf, London.

Eldridge, J., Kitzinger, J. and Williams, K. (1997) *The Mass Media and Power in Modern Britain*, Oxford University Press, Oxford.

Kitzinger, J. (1993) 'Media messages and what people know about Acquired Immune Deficiency Syndrome' in Eldridge, J. (ed.) *Getting the Message: News, Truth and Power*, Routledge, London.

Kitzinger, J. (1999) 'A sociology of media power: key issues in audience reception research' in Philo, G. (ed.) *Message Received: Glasgow Media Group Research 1993–1998*, Longman, London.

Lister, R. (1997) *Citizenship: Feminist Perspectives*, Macmillan, Basingstoke.

Marshall, T.H. (1950) *Citizenship and Social Class*, Cambridge University Press, Cambridge.

Oliver, M. (1990) *The Politics of Disablement*, Macmillan, Basingstoke.

Phillips, A. (1997) 'From inequality to difference: a severe case of displacement', *New Left Review*, 224, pp. 143–153.

Phillips, A. (1999) *Which Equalities Matter?*, Polity Press, Cambridge.

Philo, G. (ed.) (1996) *Media and Mental Distress*, Addison-Wesley, Harlow.

Riddell, S., Wilkinson, H. and Baron, S. (1998) 'From emancipatory research to focus group: people with learning difficulties and the research process' in Clough, P. and Barton, L. (eds) *Articulating with Difficulty: Research Voices in Inclusive Education*, Paul Chapman Publishing, London.

Shakespeare, T. (1994) 'Cultural representations of disabled people: dustbins for disavowal', *Disability and Society*, 9(3), pp. 283–301.

Shakespeare, T. (1996) 'Doing disability research: rules of engagement', *Disability and Society*, **11**(1), pp. 115–121.

Shakespeare, T. and Watson, N. (2001) 'Making the Difference: Disability, politics and recognition' in Albrecht, G.L., Seelman, K.D. and Bury, M. (eds) *Handbook of Disability Studies*, Sage, London.

The Report of the Commission on Social Justice (Borrie Report) (1994) *Social Justice: Strategies for National Renewal*, Vintage, London.

Thomas, C. (1999) *Female Forms: Experiencing and Understanding Disability*, Open University Press, Buckingham.

Young, I.M. (1990) *Justice and the Politics of Difference*, Princeton University Press, Princeton NJ.

CHAPTER 10

Disability and ethnicity: how young Asian disabled people make sense of their lives

Karl Atkin and Yasmin Hussain

Introduction

If debates about identity are complex, they are perhaps more so for disabled people from minority ethnic groups. They may wish to identify with different religious and cultural values to those of the wider society (Modood *et al.* 1994). The experience of disability in which they are struggling to reconcile the inability of the wider society to accommodate difference, while maintaining a positive identity, further complicates the situation (Oliver 1996). This chapter, based on a qualitative study, discusses how South Asian young people with an impairment sustain and negotiate different identity claims. We begin our account by outlining some key themes, with which we contextualise our empirical findings. We then describe our specific aims before discussing how we carried out the study. This leads us into our empirical account in which we explore the narratives of disabled young people, their parents and siblings.

Disability and ethnicity

The past twenty years have seen a shift in how disability is perceived in Western societies. The medical model, with its emphasis on individuality, rehabilitation and sense of personal tragedy, has been challenged by those who propose a more social model (see Oliver 1996), in which disability assumes meaning in relation to the workings of an unjust society (Barnes *et al.* 1999). This powerful and necessary critique, emphasising that many of the disadvantages faced by disabled people arise because of the wider society's inability to accommodate difference, has informed disabled people's political struggle for a positive identity (Corker and French 1998).

Despite its valuable and important role in asserting the rights of disabled people, the disability movement has been criticised for not recognising diversity (Stuart 1996). These criticisms, although not dismissing the basic assumptions of the social model, raise various interrelated themes around the definition and experience of disability and the role of social relationships. Some, for instance, argue for a more considered approach that recognises that disability might be only one aspect of an individual's identity. This further suggests that impairment can only be understood against what is considered as 'normal' for someone of their own age, gender and social class (Ahmad 2000). Normalcy is not a given universal and impairment needs to be seen in its social and cultural context. The implications of this are especially complex when it comes to dealing with disabled young people from minority ethnic groups. For example, independence and autonomy – central to the disability movement – represent social and cultural constructs, which may not have the same meaning among different ethnic groups (see Modood *et al.* 1994). This, of course, is part of a more dynamic process, reflecting broader changes in the experience of Asian young people living in the UK. Young people may adopt their own views seeking sustenance from different and often conflicting value systems. Outright rejection of their parents' ethnic and religious identities is, however, rare among the second generation, although partial and contingent acceptance as well as reinterpretation of some values does occur (Drury 1991).

The study

The broad aim of the research was to provide a detailed understanding of how young Asian people make sense of their disability, within the broader social context. The project used qualitative methods and analysis, based on semi-structured interviews. Such methods allow an examination of complex and contingent situations, behaviours, beliefs and interactions. A topic guide identified a number of key themes we hoped to explore during the interviews. This guide was developed from a review of the relevant literature on identity, disability and ethnicity; discussions with key informants; advice from the project advisory committee; and our own previous work on disability and chronic illness among minority ethnic families. The purpose of the interview was to get the young person, their parents and siblings to talk about disability within the broader social context with which they engaged. Rather than assume that disability would dominate their narratives, we created a more general topic guide that probed family relationships, life transitions and social networks. Complete interviews were then fully transcribed and organised according to analytical headings.

The sample came from diverse statutory and voluntary organisations in West Yorkshire and a small number from the West Midlands, as well as through 'snowballing'. 'Snowballing' was especially important because we wanted to include young people who may not be in regular contact with services. The interviews with young people were largely held at home, although seven were held at other locations at the request of the young person. We wanted our sample to include a range of physical impairments. Our concern was with the general experience of disability rather than the specific medical consequences of impairment for young people and their families. The young people included in the study had congenital and acquired physical impairments. These included cerebral palsy, multiple sclerosis, arthritis and impairments as a consequence of strokes and accidental injury.

The sample of 29 disabled young people included 16 males and 13 females. We were particularly keen to examine how disabled and non-disabled people negotiate life transitions (education, employment, possibly living away from the parental home, family formation) and therefore only included people who were aged between fifteen and thirty years old. The mean age of the sample was 25 years: 24 years for men and 26 for women. Fourteen respondents were aged between 15 and 24 years and 15 were between 25 and 30 years of age. In terms of religion, 19 young people were Muslim and ten were Sikh. The sampling frames available to us meant we failed to recruit any Hindu disabled young people. None of the young people interviewed were at school. Eight were at college, one attended university and nine were attending training courses. A further four were working. Most people lived at home with their parents. Eleven young people were married and two were divorced.

To supplement the material obtained from interviews with disabled young people, we spoke to 14 parents: five fathers and nine mothers. We negotiated access to parents through the young person and most allowed us to contact their parents. Interviews with parents helped us make sense of family life and the process of socialisation for both disabled and non-disabled offspring. Eight of these parents described themselves as Muslim and six as Sikh. We also spoke to 15 siblings: nine brothers and six sisters. The interviews, as we have seen, provided another important and comparative perspective on the process of family life. Siblings were matched to the gender of the disabled young person and those as close in age to the disabled young person as possible were chosen.

Young people, their parents and siblings were offered a choice of interviewer (in terms of both language and gender). Ten interviews were conducted in Punjabi, one in Urdu, and 47 in English. Those conducted in Punjabi and Urdu were translated into English for analysis. Two people refused to be tape-recorded and detailed notes were made of these interviews.

The inclusion of parents and siblings in the sample represented an important methodological principle, further reflecting our concern to ensure that disability did not dominate the respondents' narratives. As well as offering a comment on the young person's disability, family interviews also gave us a more general sense of cultural and religious reproduction. From this we could assess the extent to which impairment and disability influenced this process rather than attribute all the young person's experience to their impairment and experience of disability. As we shall see, social change and a re-negotiation of ethnic, religious and cultural identities occurred irrespective of impairment. Solely focusing on disabled young people's accounts would not have enabled us to draw out such comparisons.

Following accepted conventions of qualitative analysis, we took information from the transcripts and transferred it onto a map or framework, allowing comparison by theme and case. Young people's and their parents' and siblings' accounts were organised by categories and sub-categories, suggested by the topic guides as well as new categories we drew from our analysis of transcripts. In doing so, we felt it especially important to integrate the accounts of all three stakeholders. The material included under each heading reflected both the range and the frequency of respondents' views on particular issues and formed the basis of generalising their experience. This enabled a comparative analysis of different aspects and variations in experience, as well as the significance of the individuals' background in making sense of this experience. From this we defined concepts, accounted for patterns and ranges, established linkages and gave explanations.

Negotiating identities

We have argued that impairment can only be made sense of within the context of an individual's personal, cultural and social background. This is the starting point of our empirical analysis, in which we address the identification and negotiation of competing identity claims. We begin our account with a discussion of how young people make sense of their impairment and disability, before going on to discuss the importance of ethnic, cultural and religious values in the lives of these young people.

The meaning of disability for parents

Chronic and disabling conditions have an important impact on personal biography and identity (Ahmad 2000). Consequently, developing and sustaining a positive disabled identity is far from straightforward. In the first instance, parents' response to impairment affected the young persons' views about being disabled. Having a disabled child, for example, does have social and psychological consequences for parents. Many parents expressed feelings of guilt, frustration, anxiety, helplessness, isolation, notions of unfairness and resentment: common themes in the mainstream literature on family caring (Beresford 1994; Chamba et al. 1999).

Many parents viewed the birth of a disabled child as a catastrophe, difficult to comprehend as well as threatening in terms of its consequences for the child and parents. One mother said:

> At the end of the day it's the parents who have to go through it. We're constantly upset . . . We are constantly on edge.

Parents thus regarded disability as a tragedy, with implications not just for their future life but also for the child's religious and cultural identity and family life. Parents believed that disability made their children socially and morally more vulnerable, and limited their life chances. Parental concerns focused on issues such as the ability to successfully negotiate transitions they deemed 'normal' for non-disabled children: a good education; social skills; knowledge of parental religions and cultures; and assuming adult roles such as having a job and being married. Parents felt that their child's impairment presented additional barriers.

Parents' responses are perhaps not related to their ethnic background and Asian families seem to subscribe to the same negative views of disability held by white families (Barnes et al. 1999). At the same time, this is not to argue that there were no loving or fulfilling relationships between young people and their families. Families and young people tried hard to maintain positive relations and nearly all could still describe a generally loving family atmosphere. Parents were vital allies for their children. There is thus a constant tension in the parents' narratives as they try to make sense of their own sadness at having a disabled child, while at the same time wanting to ensure the best opportunities for their child. This sometimes explains why parents' strategy to overcome the disadvantages faced by the child may not always be in the young person's best interests, despite the best intentions of the parent.

As part of this tension, parents often criticised the extended family for having negative views of disability, despite them being close to the parents. To this extent, Asian communities' disabilist attitudes are no different from the general population (Katbamna 2000). This also reminds us that that the extended family is often a mixed blessing (Chamba *et al.* 1998) and sometimes oppressive, providing moral policing but little practical support (Katbamna *et al.* 2000). Families with a disabled child, for example, were not always welcome at family gatherings. Sushma's sister described a recent visit to her aunt's house:

> Everyone else is scared that she might break something and so will anticipate the worst and she went to my aunt's house the other day and everyone like, 'why did you bring her?'.

Young people and the family

Despite the good intentions of their parents, young people do have to negotiate negative views within the family. This is fundamental to their experience of disability. Young people have to frequently confront barriers and this is why many sometimes felt isolated and under-valued within the family. Some young people internalised these negative views and perhaps not surprisingly, young people felt that their parents' view of disability undermined their own confidence and made it difficult to sustain a positive self-image. Nineteen-year-old Shakeel felt different from his siblings, 'You think you've let everyone down, that you're odd'. Many young people also felt disability thus subverted 'normal' family hierarchies; the roles the disabled young person would usually be entitled to perform were passed on to non-disabled siblings. Young people resented such 'lack of respect', a term used repeatedly to describe their treatment by both family and other people. Such social diminution within the family ·sometimes reflected the marginalisation they experienced in the wider society. 'Social death', however, was rarely absolute and although highlighted at specific times, it was rarely a constant feature of their life. It should also be remembered – as we have seen – that most young people and their parents also described loving family relationships.

Over-protection was sometimes a particular tension between young people and their parents, reflecting many of the difficulties outlined above. Shakeel's mother said:

> When he is getting out of line. I still tell him off...He still keeps saying, 'I'm grown up. I'm 19. Don't tell me what to do'.

Parents, as we have seen, do feel the need to protect the child from the consequences of the impairment and are aware of the many problems their child will face during the process of 'growing up'. Children, on the other hand, often interpret their parents' actions as an over-reaction to the difficulties they face and – as they develop their own identities – may question their parents' definitions of what is in their interests. The young person often regarded parental concerns as restrictive and setting them aside from their peers. The feeling that parental restrictions were imposed rather than negotiated made it all the more difficult for the young person to accept. Nineteen-year-old Shakeel remarked 'I wish she [her mother] would back off, you know, give me more space'. Twenty-six-year-old Gurudyal described a similar problem. She said her family were very supportive, although they sometimes irritated her by worrying too much:

> I'll get angry, right, if they put me in cotton wool or something like that, if they watch me every minute.

Over-protectiveness, however, is not always a consequence of impairment and can be a common feature of most parent and child relationships (Jenks 1996). It thus seems an inevitable reaction of all parents to their child's growing sense of autonomy and independence (see Frydenberg 1997) and this reminds us how difficult it can be to separate the parents' response to impairment from their more general concerns about life transitions. The young people's narratives reflected this and many acknowledged that their impairment might not be the only reason for their parents' response. Some of the young people, for example, felt their parents were adopting a natural response to the dangers of 'growing up' in the late twentieth century, parents had similar concerns for their other children. This is why gender comes to inform the parents' response to their children's negotiation of independence as much as impairment. We will return to this later in the chapter.

The social meaning of disability

The negative views of disability encountered in the family could be compounded by the negative experience of broader social relationships that also tended to devalue the young people as disabled people. This is another fundamental aspect of the experience of disability and a powerful influence on how they made sense of their lives. Twenty-year-old Washeed's account was typical:

> I mean I am not an able-bodied person but I don't feel bad about that. You know I feel that they [other people] treat you, they make your life, just a little bit harder than actually what it is.

A more positive disabled identity can offer a form of pride, resistance and mobilisation and help counter such negative views. Contact with disabled people, as well as exposure to disability politics, could help counter these problems. Twenty-eight-year-old Gurupal reflected on disadvantage:

> There's a lot of talented disabled people, who have got the ability to work and I think it's important that we're given the opportunity to showcase our abilities ... I don't think of myself as disabled. It's society who's disabled by not enabling me to do this stuff. The most difficulty I experienced is through not being able to access buildings properly, not being able to get where I want to go because the facilities are not there to cater for me, so that's where I experience more discrimination really.

Few young people, however, became exposed to such social networks and many were isolated, further emphasising their sense of difference and confirming negative values of disability. As Gurubax observed: 'What is the point in getting up in the morning, when you've got nowhere to go?'

More general social networks can be important in confirming their sense of being a young person, in which they can identify with the popular images of fashion, entertainment and other symbols of youth culture as well as the mundane realties of school, employment, home life and social networks. This also offers the context in which life transitions associated with being a young person occur. To this extent, disability has to be seen within the broader context of the normative assumptions of 'being a young person'. We will return to this again when we discuss ethnicity and cultural identification. Nonetheless, this is another reminder that disability is not the only aspect of a person's identity, just as the family is more than a framework with which to engage with disability. Social networks could help support a positive self-image, reinforcing contacts with the wider society. To this extent, associating with other young people was fundamental to the young person's narratives rather than associating with young people with an impairment. Again, however, impairment could restrict the opportunities of such encounters and further contribute to the young person's sense of isolation. Nineteen-year-old Shakeel was asked about what he did with his spare time and his response summed up the feelings of many other disabled young people: 'Spare time? I think every day is spare time for me'.

Nasira similarly found it difficult to make friends:

> I don't have any friends because I don't go anywhere... They don't want to come round because I'm disabled, you see, they don't want to know me.

This contrasted with the experience of their non-disabled siblings, who, by and large, had wider social networks and more frequent engagement with such networks.

Ethnic, cultural and religious identification

A positive disabled identity can embody specific eurocentric assumptions and as such fails to offer a framework with which the young person can celebrate the ethnic, religious and cultural identity. Of immediate concern is the possibility of the social model becoming an extension of the dominant white culture and undermining cultural, religious and ethnic values (see Ahmad *et al.* 1998). Independence and autonomy represent social and cultural constructs, which may not have the same meaning among different ethnic groups. The sense of independence of young Asian people in the UK is informed by how they make sense of their ethnic and religious culture within the broader British culture to which they are also exposed (see Modood *et al.* 1994). This is why establishing autonomy and independence, although as important to Asian young people living in the UK as their 'white' counterparts, can assume different connotations (Atkin and Ahmad 2001). The narratives of young people and their non-disabled siblings reflect this. Developing and sustaining an identity separate from their parents and exercising some control over their own lives, for example, is not always equated with leaving home and establishing an independent existence (see also Ahmad 2000). Asian disabled young people have to balance the need to exercise control over their lives with a sense of mutuality, interdependence and ability to reciprocate.

This discussion of independence further reminds us that as well as negotiating the meaning of disability, young people may also wish to celebrate their ethnic, cultural and religious difference. This, as we have seen, becomes important both in terms of their experience of disability but also in its own right, as an important marker of social identity. Further, such identifications become especially salient in terms of the presumed predicament of the 'second generation', irrespective of whether they have an impairment. Academic policy and lay discourses tend to over-emphasise 'cultural conflict' between young people and their parents, thus racialising the routine negotiation of values and behaviours between generations (see Brah 1992). And although generational change is observed within South Asian communities, outright rejection of ethnic and religious identities remains rare in the second generation. Literature on inter-generational relations presents a picture of cultural retention and successful negotiation of identities. Does impairment, however, compromise this and in turn, to what extent does ethnic, religious and cultural identification further mediate the experience of disability?

As a starting point, defining ethnicity is a far from neutral exercise and the term embodies such notions as language, culture, religion, nationality, and a shared heritage (Fenton 1999; Modood *et al.* 1994). Ethnicity is increasingly recognised as a political symbol; one which defines not just exclusion by a powerful majority but also self-identification as a symbol of belonging, pride and mobilisation (Werbner 1990). It is, therefore, important to break down its significance and meaning to the young person.

Contact with parental country of origin is an important symbol of ethnic identification (Basit 1997; Modood *et al.* 1997). Links are cemented and reinvented through visits, remittances, transfer of cultural goods, foodstuffs and clothes, and marriages between young people in Britain and in countries of origin (Modood *et al.* 1997). Impairment can mediate all these links, although young people also share similar views to their siblings and in turn express similar ambivalences to other South Asian people living in the UK. Gurbax's brother, for example, did not share any particular links to his parent's homeland, India: 'I come from here'. Gurbax shared this view.

Ethnic identification remained ambivalent at two levels. First, as many young people identified with being British as with being Pakistani or Indian. Minority ethnic people's adoption of English or British identities remains complex; such claims are sometimes difficult to sustain because of the racialised nature of British identity with Britishness carrying notions of European heritage, white colour and a colonial past (Ahmad and Husband 1993). However, young people – both those with an impairment and their non-disabled siblings – challenged such racialised constructions of Britishness. Their sense of Britishness was often a pragmatic reflection of being born and living in Britain. Mushtaq's sibling said, 'England's my country really, just here, I'm used to here and everything'. Disabled young people, however, found identification with Britishness particularly meaningful, an argument which relates closely to being disabled and being accorded more 'respect' within British than Pakistani contexts. For our respondents, the reservations and negative experiences we outline above perhaps enhance the young people's sense of Britishness. Britishness was regarded as being more disabled-friendly and offering opportunities and respect for disabled people. To this extent, impairment can influence the young person's sense of 'ethnicity'.

Religious and cultural identification

Lived religion is often impossible to differentiate from ethnic cultural mores and expectations (Ahmed 1988; Ahmed 1992). Nonetheless religion can offer a fundamental form of identification for South Asian young people living in the UK. However, young people did not have the same access to religious and cultural socialisation as their non-disabled siblings (see also Chamba *et al.* 1998; Ahmad *et al.* 1998). Nineteen-year-old Tahir does not know much about religion and he contrasts his knowledge to that of his brothers who are able to read the Qur'an and attend the Mosque: 'I don't go to the Mosque because I'm disabled and they don't teach me nothing'.

Young people, as we have seen, had poor access to wider community networks. Many felt isolated and estranged from their own communities. A particular problem was religious education and the role of mosques and temples. The emphasis on rote learning in mosques and temples, the total reliance on another spoken language (usually Urdu) and the teachers' lack of acknowledgement of the disabled young person's needs did little to enthuse young people about religious education. Parents bemoaned their children's lack of religious understanding and observance; those whose children had acquired such understanding against the odds reported this with pride. Their concerns were partly justified. Relatively few respondents had a sophisticated understanding of their religion, or the cross-cutting of religious and ethnic values. This contrasts with their siblings and possibly their non-disabled peers, who may have a more sophisticated understanding of religious and cultural traditions, and may be better equipped to use these as flexible resources (Drury 1991; Ahmad *et al.* 1998; Basit 1997).

Nonetheless it is important to see this within a broader context. No young person was totally detached from their parents' ethnic, religious and cultural traditions. This is not to argue, as we have seen, that they had no religious or cultural awareness, or that all young people faced this problem. Despite these disadvantages, most young people managed to acquire a working knowledge of religious and cultural traditions and identified with their family religion and ethnicity. A few demonstrated a sophisticated understanding of how religious and ethnic traditions intersect and used these arguments to challenge parental perspectives or expectations. Most young people knew enough about their religious and cultural values both to feel they belonged to their religious community and to behave 'appropriately' – examples include knowledge of culturally appropriate gender roles and rules about foods. However, conflicts did arise, although these were more a consequence of interpretation of cultural values rather than of a lack of knowledge. Partly these were over definitions of religious and cultural restrictions. Some young people challenged parental restrictions about codes of dress, for example, by arguing that these were based on ethnic culture and not on religious values; these claims were used to argue for concessions. Fatima (aged 28) knows she should maintain her modesty, but said this could be done with either 'traditional' or Western clothes. Her parents were happy with this and Fatima successfully addressed their concerns:

No, I mean my mum and dad, they prefer if we wore traditional clothes at home, but if we're going out to work, or going to college or university, they've never stopped us wearing trousers. But that doesn't mean we'd go and wear short skirts, things, you know show our legs, sort of things. As long as we're covered, they don't mind. Otherwise, I think they would get too upset, my family.

The separation of an idealised notion of Islam from lived religion is an important tool for seeking concessions (Mumtaz and Shaheed 1987; Ahmed 1988). These arguments implicated parental countries of origin with which many respondents, as we have seen, had an ambivalent relationship. This reflects a wider process, from which disabled Asian young people do not seem isolated. Religion has risen in importance as a symbol of identification and mobilisation in recent years (Ahmed and Donnon 1994; Samad 1992). The decline of class- and colour-based analysis and mobilisation in relation to ethnic and race relations has gone hand-in-hand with an increasing recognition of the significance of cultural and religious identifications (Samad 1992). In particular, there has been a re-imagining of Islam as a global religion, stripped of its ethnic identifications (Ahmed and Donnon 1994).

Socialisation into cultural and religious values, against the backdrop of a potentially hostile majority culture, is a major concern of minority ethnic groups (Anthias 1992; Modood et al. 1994; Ahmad 1996). Disability as we have seen can hinder routine socialisation. Equally, the possible greater freedoms afforded to some disabled children, introduces them to influences many parents would wish to guard their children against (see Ahmad 1996). Perceptions of new freedoms as threatening prized cultural values, such as parental authority, possible changes in marriage choices and concerns about sexual permissiveness are held strongly by the older generation of Asian people (Modood et al. 1994). Nonetheless, it should be emphasised that this occurs irrespective of impairment.

Most young people and parents, irrespective of disability, employ various strategies to avoid conflict (Drury 1991; Afshar and Maynard 1994; Modood et al. 1994). This is usually done through using particular and flexible interpretations of cultural rules, employing different cultural symbols to counter particular arguments, and avoiding open displays of behaviours which would cause offence. For example, a woman, as we have seen, may use her identity as a 'Muslim woman' to challenge restrictions, which, she argues, are located in 'ethnic culture'. People negotiate 'deviant' behaviour against the backdrop of normative assumptions by emphasising the unique features of their situation, giving a legitimate excuse to contravene norms without damaging identities or severing relationships (Finch and Mason 1994). Such negotiations of behaviour, if they are not to irreparably damage one's social or moral identity, require cultural understanding and social skills. Not having full access to this understanding could cause problems. Having an impairment, as we have seen, can have an impact on this, but its influence is not absolute and young people do seem to have sufficient cultural capital to negotiate these various influences on their lives, without being confrontational. To this extent, their experience shares some similarities with their non-disabled peers.

Young female respondents, for example, had a strong relationship to youth culture, but often within the context of religious and cultural identifications. Wearing smart and fashionable clothes was important as was an interest in music and friendships. However, being trendy was not always equated with being westernised. Many talked about Asian fashionable clothes – Indian films, Asian satellite television, Asian clothes shops and fashion magazines all provide visions of 'coolness' and being fashionable. Some took part in making appropriate clothes at home. Western dress, for some young disabled female respondents and families, was also deemed to be at odds with requirements of modesty and honour. Their non-disabled siblings shared this perception.

Gender, more generally, played an important part in how parents responded to their disabled children's social relationship. This again, however, needs to be seen within the wider context. Families' response to gender occurred irrespective of impairment and non-disabled female siblings complained of similar restrictions. The protection of moral identities is fundamental to understanding this. Nonetheless, impairment further mediated the families' sense of gender relationships. Most parents, as we have seen, felt disability made their children vulnerable. Parents responded differently to young men and women because of the gendered nature of moral identities. Muslim, Hindu and Sikh parents shared these views. Young disabled men were afforded greater concessions, almost as a compensation for being disabled, than their non-disabled peers. Conversely, perceived threats to young disabled women's moral identities were countered by resisting their incursions into the wider social world. Female moral identities are perceived as being more easily damaged and less easy to repair within South Asian communities, having consequences for the individual and the family and affecting marriage prospects (Wilson 1979; Mumtaz and Shaheed 1987; Katbamna *et al.* 2000). While one can bemoan the sexism of these normative values, their consequences for the families and young people are real and serious.

Most young people respected their parents' views but some young women – irrespective of impairment – were beginning to voice criticisms and commented on the unfairness of such differential treatment. Twenty-eight-year-old Fatima said her parents keep a closer eye on her because she is a woman. Her disabled brother had more freedom:

> My brother's got no pressure at all, I mean he comes in and out, it's like you don't even know where he is, he could be anywhere. Whereas I go away for minute and they want to know where you are.

As well as offering a form of self-identification, a symbol of belonging, pride and mobilisation (Samad 1992), culture can also have a wider political significance, defining minority groups in relation to a powerful majority. We have already touched on this when we discussed the concerns of parents about 'new freedoms'. A sense of difference, enforced by racism and discrimination thus remains an important influence in how South Asian young people make sense of their lives. Substantive citizenship rights are often denied to minority ethnic groups as they are to disabled people (Husband 1996). Racism can, therefore, continue to inform young people's sense of identity. To a large extent this occurred irrespective of impairment.

Racism was also manifest in the unwillingness of services to provide appropriate and accessible support. Institutional racism is fundamental in explaining this (Ahmad 2000). Minority ethnic people, for example, often find their needs located in their own supposed failings. They were excluded from services on the basis of language, experienced insensitivity to cultural diversity and were subject to myths and stereotypes that denied them the support they need (Ahmad and Atkin 1996). Young people and their families' narratives reflected this. There was also a sense, however, that the young person's impairment added to their sense of discrimination. At its most straightforward, disabled people – irrespective of ethnicity – experience problems in accessing provision. This, however, is not a simple practical problem but embodies specific assumptions about disability, which challenge the way in which disabled people can exercise control over their lives (Priestley 1999). Professional help, under the guise of 'benevolent' intervention is often geared towards 'rehabilitation', which undermines the voice of disabled people (Corker and French 1998). This can further increases their sense of isolation and makes it difficult to sustain a positive sense of their disability.

Generally, barriers, a consequence of both racism and disablism, mean that Asian disabled young people have difficulties in having their needs recognised and acted upon by the welfare state. This failure to respect diversity not only creates practical difficulties but also mediates the young person's sense of selfhood (Jones *et al.* 2001).

Discussion

Current debates about ethnicity and disability tend to argue that certain identities and forms of oppression are more authentic than others. The political mobilisation around 'disabled' identities privileges these definitions of selfhood over others (see Oliver 1996). There is no doubt that disability was a powerful influence on how young Asian people made sense of their lives. To this extent, young people had to deal with negative views about their impairment, both from their family as well as the wider society. It also mediated their sense of ethnic, religious and cultural identity. Privileging disabled identity, however, is an unhelpful starting point in discussing how young Asian disabled people make sense of their lives. This does not deny the relevance of the social model of disability, which has been tremendously influential in asserting a more positive definition of disability. Nonetheless, the social model has been slow in responding to diversity (Ahmad 2000) and this has led minority ethnic disabled writers to focus on the neglect of 'race' in disability politics (Hill 1993; Stuart 1996).

This suggests some redefinition of the social model is required and, in response to this, we have argued that impairment can only be made sense of within the context of an individual's personal, cultural and social diversity. As we have seen, our respondents had multiple identifications, some held more strongly than others, and many becoming particularly salient in certain circumstances or places. To this extent, South Asian young people with an impairment potentially have a number of identity claims in relation to ethnicity, culture, religion, youth and disability. Disability is an important influence in the way they make sense of their lives, but this does not occur within a vacuum. As many have argued, identities can only be made sense of as a complex and dynamic interplay between agency and structure (see Bourdieu 1977 and Giddens 1991).

Discussing identities with these young people was a complex undertaking; a task which may well have proved impossible without the use of flexible tools and methods. And yet, all had something to say on the topic. Identities were not so closely tied to single issues or symbols that an individual could only be one thing; young people held multiple identifications, some more strongly than others, and used these flexibly in different situations. Identifications also demonstrated hybridity, a variety of historical, international, ideological and political factors influencing their sense of selfhood and relationship with others. It is not a question of forsaking one claim for another and choosing between a 'Western' or 'Asian' way of life (Modood *et al.* 1994). Young people need to find space to express a variety of different and competing identity claims. Further, these identifications were far from ethereal, disconnected to questions of power, structure and history. Structures and resources were closely tied to people assuming or discarding particular identities. Both racism and disabilism were important influences in young people's sense of identity.

To conclude, exploring identities is a difficult undertaking, especially when identity claims are so numerous and contested as in our study. Our study offers no support to notions of singular identities or of a hierarchy of identifications. Our work shows that identity claims of disabled young people were negotiated and contingent, allowing freedoms within contexts in which ethnicity, religion, gender, social status, racism, generational relations and the meaning of being disabled were important considerations. And although our sample was largely composed of Pakistani Muslim respondents, the group of Hindu and Sikh respondents[1] reported similar experiences and perspectives, suggesting that the findings may apply to South Asian groups more generally.

Acknowledgements

This research was funded by the Joseph Rowntree Foundation. Our thanks go to the families for their time and the many professionals who helped us get in touch with these families. A special thanks goes to the project advisory committee, for its encouragement and support. Waqar Ahmed provided helpful comments on previous drafts of this chapter.

[1] Several Hindu disabled people were recruited to the study but, after initially agreeing to be interviewed, decided not to take part. They did, however, give us permission to talk to their parents.

References

Afshar, H. and Maynard, M. (1994) *The dynamics of 'race' and gender*, Taylor and Francis, London.

Ahmad, W.I.U. (1996) 'Family obligations and social change in Asian families' in Ahmad, W.I.U. and Atkin, K. (eds) *'Race' and community care*, Open University Press, Buckingham.

Ahmad, W.I.U. (2000) *Ethnicity, Disability and Chronic Illness*, Open University Press, Buckingham.

Ahmad, W.I.U. and Atkin, K. (1996) *'Race' and community care*, Open University Press, Buckingham.

Ahmad, W.I.U., Darr, A., Jones, L. and Nisar, G. (1998) *Deafness and Ethnicity*, Policy Press, Bristol.

Ahmad, W.I.U. and Husband, C. (1993) 'Religious identity, citizenship and welfare: the case of Muslims in Britain', *American Journal of Islamic Social Science*, 10(2), pp. 217–233.

Ahmed, A.S. (1988) *Discovering Islam: Making Sense of Muslim History and Society*, Routledge, London.

Ahmed, A.S. and Donnon, H. (1994) *Islam, Globalisation and Identity*, Routledge, London.

Ahmed, L. (1992) *Women and Gender in Islam*, Yale University Press, New Haven, CT and London.

Anthias, F. (1992) *Ethnicity, Class, Gender and Migration*, Avebury, Aldershot.

Atkin, K. and Ahmad, W.I.U. (2000) 'Living with a sickle cell disorder: how young people negotiate their care and treatment' in Ahmad, W.I.U. (ed.) *Ethnicity, disability and chronic Illness*, Open University Press, Buckingham.

Atkin, K. and Ahmad, W.I.U. (2001) 'Living a "normal" life: how young people cope with thalassaemia major or sickle cell disorder', *Social Science and Medicine*, **53**, pp. 615–626.

Barnes, C., Mercer, G. and Shakespeare, T. (1999) *Exploring disability: a sociological introduction*, Polity Press, Cambridge.

Basit, T.N. (1997) *Eastern Values, Western Milieu: Identities and Aspirations of Adolescent British Muslim Girls*, Ashgate, Aldershot.

Beresford, B. (1994) *Expert opinions: a national survey of parents caring for a severely disabled child*, Policy Press, Bristol.

Bourdieu, P. (1977) *Outline of a Theory of Practice*, Cambridge University Press, Cambridge.

Brah, A. (1992) 'Women of South Asian origin in Britain' in Braham, P., Rattansi, A. and Skellington, R. (eds) *Racism and anti-racism: inequalities, opportunities and policies*, Sage, London.

Chamba, R., Ahmad, W.I.U. and Jones, L. (1998) *Improving Services for Asian Deaf Children*, Policy Press, Bristol.

Chamba, R., Hirst, M., Lawton, D., Ahmad, W. and Beresford, B. (1999) *Expert voices: A national survey of minority ethnic parents caring for a severely disabled child*, Policy Press, Bristol.

Corker, M. and French, S. (1998) *Disability discourse*, Open University Press, Buckingham.

Drury, B. (1991) 'Sikh girls and the maintenance of ethnic culture', *New Community*, **17**(3), pp. 387–99.

Fenton, S. (1999) *Ethnicity: Racism, Class and Culture*, Macmillan, Basingstoke.

Finch, J. and Mason, J. (1994) *Negotiating family responsibilities*, Routledge, London.

Finklestein, V. (1993) 'The commonality of disability' in Swain, J., Finklestein, V., French, S. and Oliver, M. (eds) *Disabling Barriers – Enabling Environments*, Sage, London.

Frydenberg, E. (1997) *Adolescent coping: theoretical and research perspectives*, Routledge, London.

Giddens, A. (1991) *Modernity and Self-Identity*, Routledge, London.

Hill, M. (1993) 'They're not our brothers: the disability movement and the black disability movement' in Begum, N., Hill, M. and Stevens, A. (eds) *Reflections: Views of Black Disabled People on Their Lives and Community Care*, CCETSW, London.

Husband, C. (1996) 'Defining and containing diversity: community, ethnicity and citizenship' in Ahmad, W.I.U. and Atkin, K. (eds) *'Race' and community care*, Open University Press, Buckingham.

Jenks, C. (1996) *Childhood*, Routledge, London.

Jones, L., Atkin, K. and Ahmad, W.I.U. (2001) 'Supporting Asian Deaf young people and their families: The role of professionals and services', *Disability and Society*, **16**(1), pp. 51–70.

Katbamna, S., Bhakta, P. and Parker, G. (2000) 'Perceptions of disability and care-giving relationships among South Asian Communities' in Ahmad, W.I.U. (ed.) *Ethnicity, disability and chronic illness*, Open University Press, Buckingham.

Modood, T., Beishon, S. and Virdee, S. (1994) *Changing Ethnic Identities*, Policy Studies Institute, London.

Modood, T., Berthoud, R., Lakey, J., Nazroo, J., Smith, P., Virdee, S. and Beishon, S. (1997) *Ethnic Minorities in Britain: Diversity and Disadvantage* (Fourth PSI Survey), Policy Studies Institute, London.

Mumtaz, K. and Shaheed, F. (1987) *Women of Pakistan*, Zed, London.

Oliver, M. (1996) *Understanding disability: from theory to practice*, Macmillan, Basingstoke.

Priestley, M. (1999) *Disability, politics and community care*, Jessica Kingsley, London.

Samad, Y. (1992) 'Book burning and race relations: political mobilisation of Bradford Muslims', *New Community*, **18**(4), pp. 507–19.

Stuart, O. (1996) 'Yes, we mean black disabled people too' in Ahmad, W.I.U. and Atkin, K. (eds) *'Race' and Community Care*, Open University Press, Buckingham.

Werbner, P. (1990) *The Migration Process: Capital, Gifts and Offerings among British Pakistanis*, Berg, London.

Wilson, A. (1979) *Finding a Voice: South Asian Women in Britain*, Virago, London.

CHAPTER 11

Can multiculturalism encompass disability?

Andrew Jakubowicz and Helen Meekosha

Introduction

How do disability culture and the cultural experiences of people with disabilities fit into ideas about cultural diversity? This chapter uses the experience of settler societies in general, and Australia in particular, to explore the discursive turmoil generated when disability meets multiculturalism. Our aim is to elucidate what disability culture might involve, and then interrogate multiculturalism through a disability lens. The end point would be a way of thinking about cultural diversity which valorises disability as a dimension of normal difference in pluralist societies.

Settler societies resulting from the imperial eras of the European metropolitan powers, were all faced with a series of challenges in their struggle to assert the dominance of their settler elites. The initial struggle involved war with the Indigenous people, the expropriation of their lands, and the suppression of their cultures. These wars resulted in marginalised populations, who are still experiencing the residue of their encounters, and all of which show high levels of disability. The populations that were then imported – through slavery and/or immigration – went on to form what have been described as multicultural societies; that is, societies characterised by cultural differences that are managed within a single social order. The control of population inflows has become a major role of the nation state. Within these societies the state has been concerned to ensure the 'quality' of its population, through hygienist ideologies of selection and breeding, and ideologies which justify the hegemony of the elite. The confluence of these elements provides the terrain on which this chapter is built.

Two questions then apply – what are the processes through which individual identity is formed and given sustenance, and what are the conditions under which recognition of cultures can occur? These questions require an understanding of the political economy of disability in culturally diverse societies.

When Pakistani refugee Shahraz Kayani poured petrol on himself and ignited it at the doors of Australia's national parliament early in 2001 (he later died of his injuries), the nation was suddenly awakened to the reality of its population policy – one which accepted able-bodied refugees but rejected those with disabilities likely to be a cost to the community. The Australian Attorney General defended the government's refusal to allow the man's daughter with cerebral palsy to enter the country (the trigger for his self-immolation), on the grounds that:

certain health criteria must be met by all visa applicants in order to protect Australia's public health, contain expenditure in health and community service budgets, and protect the access of Australians to scarce medical resources... (Williams 2001)

The Attorney went on to claim that:

Australia is a country to which people with disabilities can, and do, migrate – and Australia enjoys their contribution. If there is a message to be drawn from this, it would seem to be a positive one. (ibid.)

The positive aspects of the message were clear to the Attorney, but few others could find in this tragedy much to celebrate. However there is as yet barely any public awakening to the relation between disability and racism in government policy.

The disability movement has been involved in a struggle for recognition within the political, intellectual and cultural milieu of contemporary Australian society. Yet there is little sense in the wider society of the processes of reconciliation necessary to resolve the broken lives and families of many people with disabilities. This unselfconscious exclusion has become widespread in cultural studies and too widespread in progressive politics.

A new National Museum of Australia opened in March 2001, claiming to reflect the diversity of Australian society. In its introductory multimedia environment, *Circa*, it seeks to present a series of images and voices of Australia – rural and urban, old and young, Indigenous and immigrant, traditional and *avant garde*, male and female, gay and straight, wealthy and poor, and almost every other duality to be imagined. Except that there were no people with apparent disabilities in the 12-minute exposition. Indeed in the whole museum there appear to be only three references to disability – two are of women who are known as minor cultural celebrities; one is an anthropological recording of the Indigenous Wik people dancing a story of a young boy made into a cripple (*sic*) by the spirits, for some cultural transgression.

This difficulty that cultural institutions have in understanding issues associated with disability and culture, can be summarised as:

▦ a problem in conceptualisation of the 'audience' for cultural ideas, who are assumed to be able-bodied;

▦ a problem in the conceptualisation of the multicultural/cultural agenda, which provides no place for disability;

▦ a problem in the theorisation of social and cultural relations, which fails to problematise the body as a social construct in a political realm of normalising practices;

▦ difficulty in understanding the links between disability and racialised oppression, despite the example of the Third Reich in its inexorable march from the eradication of 'less than German people' with disabilities to the eradication of people from the 'less than human races'.

⬤ Critical multiculturalism and the problem of the able body

It is particularly appropriate then that the terrain of the multicultural debate be critiqued from a disability perspective. Cultural studies that exclude consideration of bodily capacity and the lived experience of different bodily incarnations cannot claim to offer an adequate theoretical armoury. Cultural theory that ignores the advances made in disability theory significantly limits itself when trying to offer explanations and analyses of contemporary social relations.

Multiculturalism and multicultural theory have developed as philosophical and policy frameworks for interpreting and managing cultural diversity, usually labelled as 'racial' or ethnic. These categories encompass differences of physical appearance (ascribed to 'race'), language, religion, norms and beliefs, and national or regional origins. Multiculturalism has been a portmanteau term, which can be unpacked to reflect specific ideological assumptions and programmatic outcomes. McLaren (1994) has suggested that multiculturalism can be variously perceived as:

- a corporate strategy of inclusion of subordinate cultures in hierarchies of difference (e.g. multicultural marketing, productive diversity),

- a liberal strategy concerned with facilitating access equal to that available to dominant groups (e.g. access and equity),

- a left-liberal approach that validates all cultures equally irrespective of content (e.g. anti-racist strategies), and

- a critical multiculturalism that problematises the concept of culture as a discrete collectivity of social practices (e.g. 'white' theory, theories of hybridity).

We will deal here primarily with critical multiculturalism, as it provides some useful pointers to readings of policy and practice for disability theory. The wider debates about diversity are important in the particular issues raised in this chapter. Fraser (1995) has argued that the redistributive agendas in the struggles by subaltern groups have been overcome by the rise of identity politics. In essence, the political goals of redistributive justice sought on the basis of membership of a particular category (e.g. women, ethnic minority etc.), have been lost in the demand for cultural recognition and alternative cultural spaces. Others (Young 1997) have argued that cultural recognition is crucial to gaining economic rights – that is, if you have no cultural validity you cannot gain purchase on the system which reallocates economic benefits. Out of this argument has arisen the notion of 'bi-valency', the understanding of the complex interrelationship between economic and cultural practice.

Multiculturalism has been challenged to incorporate both a redistributive agenda (in terms of economic and material outcomes for defined groups), and an identity and cultural difference agenda (in terms of affirmation of communal self-definitions). Traditions in the field have tended to keep these dimensions apart, so that redistributive arguments have focused on the sphere of income and wealth inequality, employment opportunities, the ghettoisation of communities, and the specific gendered experience of subaltern communities.

The influence of cultural studies can be found in the exploration of questions of hybridity and identity, the emergence of the concept of 'diaspora' to indicate a point of authentic origins for historically dispersed communities, and the interrogation of the politics of speaking position, as in the issue of the 'White voice'. There is now recognition that cultures are fluid, ever forming and reforming constellations, in which individuals are differentiated from each other, and from which relations of super- and sub-ordination can be inflected in many directions – not only by race/ethnicity, but by class, gender, age, subculture, sexuality and locality. Thus multiculturalism can move either towards an examination of the magnitude of cultural porosity in an unproblematised able-bodied world, or towards a recognition of the problematic status of the 'able' body. In the latter case, we would be able to examine both the cultural frames through which disability is constituted and interpreted across different cultures, and the nature of disability cultures within wider social environments. Of particular interest are the similarities between approaches to Whiteness, and approaches to Able-bodiedness in postcolonial and disability theories.

Multicultural theory and disability theory come together in their common concerns for the politics of recognition, the politics of redistribution, and the conceptualisation of a social relations model of cultural expression (Gilson and Depoy 2000). In the work of writers such as Honneth (1995), society and individual identity are formed in parallel through constantly reinforced networks of reciprocal recognition of social presence, and thereby of the right to participate in the defining of social agendas and cultural directions. Mutual recognition is a precondition for the realisation of the self and the development of individual identity and self-esteem. Taylor's (1994) argument in relation to multiculturalism points to the dialogic nature of social relations, and the critical role played by positive recognition in the development of an undamaged identity. The relational model of identity allows an understanding of inter-cultural relations that includes all cultures as realms of equal moral standing. The damage done by non-recognition lies in the erosion of identity and self-confidence, and thereby the undermining of the possibilities of inter-subjective validation.

Disability can be understood using these analytical approaches, and starting from an awareness of the community as already ability-diverse. In order to develop this argument, we need first to demonstrate the importance of disability studies as a theoretical field and the intellectual buttress for a political practice; and second, to explore how disability studies can influence the field of multicultural studies and the political practices associated with it.

Australia – a diverse settler society in crisis

Over the past decade the idea of Australia as a pluralist society which saw itself in government rhetoric composed of many different and equally legitimate interest groups, has been overwhelmed by a political project that has portrayed society as comprising a legitimate, homogenous and superior cultural core, under attack from illegitimate divergent cultural special interests. This view, most clearly advocated by the conservative (Liberal Party) Prime Minister John Howard, has promoted the sense of a 'true' culture, with its roots in a white and essentially 'Anglo-Celtic' heritage, standing at the apex of a cultural pyramid. The way forward for society, he has suggested, lies in the internalisation of these core values, and the abandonment or at least subordination of alternative values and cultural practices. While there are many contradictions in the presentation of these assumed core values (for instance, they are not at times very different from the 'Asian values' advocated by critics of Australia such as Malaysia's Dr Mahatir), the impact of the argument is to reduce the recognition of difference, and thereby the legitimacy of claims made by the denigrated 'special interests'.

The first onslaught on pluralism focused, as many commentators have noted, on multiculturalism and ethnic group rights – the closure of the Office of Multicultural Affairs, the Bureau for Immigration, Multicultural and Population Research, and the cutbacks to the Human Rights and Equal Opportunity Commission. This was accompanied by systematic restrictions on the rights of refugees, and the establishment of a string of concentration camps in which refugees, mainly from the Middle East, were and are kept in social isolation, physical discomfort and under conditions of bureaucratic intimidation. At the same time most of the key national women's organisations were 'de-funded', and most were forced to reduce their activities to a very low level.

More dramatically still, the Indigenous project which flourished after the legal victory of the Mir people in 1992 (the Mabo case) was attacked, with the imposition of the so-called 'Ten-point Plan' to reduce Indigenous rights for land and cultural autonomy (Brace 2000). More recently the concept of Mutual Obligation has been advanced as a means of rolling back welfare rights, and currently, Mutual Obligation (McClure 2000) is being assessed as a means of reducing access to disability rights. Overall, the access to basic support services has declined for people with disabilities, while the prison system has become a *de facto* public housing environment for many people with developmental and psychiatric disabilities (Disability Council of New South Wales 2000). The Australian situation indicates the broad agenda of conservative derecognition of social movements; yet these social movements themselves have not necessarily acknowledged the normalising practices that may be common to the experiences of all subaltern bodies.

● Culture – the dimension of social meanings

Disability studies with its direct challenge to theories of alterity, subaltern status and ideologies of domination, opens up ways of examining cultural diversity that cannot otherwise be approached. Viewed from a disability-sensitive perspective, multicultural studies can be interrogated. Critical questions about the embodied expression of social hierarchies can be confronted. Given that national population policies and worldviews underpin both multicultural and disability practices, an analysis which recognises this commonality seems overdue. Multiculturalism as a diverse set of discourses of difference has also been subject to critical appraisal – as a set of categorical projects that ultimately fail to account for complex and fluid identities, and changing power relations.

Meanwhile, Disability Studies has emerged over the past twenty years or so as a theoretical area developed in antagonism to the previous dominant paradigms (social order, medical and rehabilitative) which had sought to manage people with disabilities and their social relations. In simple terms, modernity had seen the development of various related forms of disciplinary regimes (Foucault 1994). Initially regimentation of the body and then manipulation of the mind characterised control strategies in society. Disability, which is the social relationship imposed on people with impairments by the wider society, was constituted through segregation on the one hand, and medical and psychiatric intervention on the other.

Throughout the nineteenth and early twentieth centuries in western societies, those defined as handicapped or crippled were taken from their families of origin, and incarcerated in increasingly constraining environments, such as asylums, long-term hospitals and other institutions. By the early twentieth century the separation of the current generation was complemented by active intervention to prevent reproduction – usually through sterilisation. In the USA the American Eugenics Movement had no difficulty in linking disability with immigration – seeking to exclude less aesthetically desirable immigrants, while sterilising those within the country who might give birth to unattractive impaired children, and allowing 'defective' babies to die (Pernick 1997).

By the late 1930s eugenicist ideologies based on aesthetic and moral hierarchies, were used to rationalise the active termination of the lives of the current generation as well – most vigorously in Nazi Germany and Austria. There, the murder of impaired citizens preceded and prefigured the murder of politically and then racially defined outsiders. Disability was the proving ground for the Holocaust, though this dimension has not been well researched or understood (Rozen 1999).

Medical approaches to disability expanded throughout the post-war period, where scientific interpretations of disability gained strength. Increasingly the person with impairments was defined by their condition, and the institutional response became to 'cure' the condition, prevent it (especially through genetic screening and abortion), or suppress its manifestations through medication and seclusion. While folk models of disability persisted (expressed in terms of personal failing or tragedy), the concentration on the individual (and perhaps the immediate family) directed attention away from the wider social processes.

These wider processes were expressed in two broad dimensions – a concern to modify the behaviour of the impaired person to reduce the socially disabling responses (known initially as 'normalisation' and given practical form in the PASSING programs of US disability theorist Wolf Wolfensberger (Wolfensberger 1983)); and the complete opposite, the emphasis on the rights of the individual to full social participation on as close as possible their own terms (Nirje 1985). It was in this context that the social model of disability was fashioned, and the idea of disability studies took form.

The Social Model – especially in its British expression in the work of disability activist scholars such as Finkelstein (1988), Barton (1993, 1994), Barnes (Barnes *et al.* 1999) and Oliver (1996) – drew heavily on social constructionist paradigms of the social realm, and the practical experience of political change. The paradigm argued that disability was a social construct, a systematic pattern of oppression, produced by 'disabling societies', through failure to modify social arrangements to lessen barriers to access by people with impairments. Its underlying thesis argued that societies had to change the way they perceived 'disabled people', through overcoming disabling attitudes, and ensuring equality of access for people with disabilities – in education, employment, housing, transport, cultural expression, social interaction and personal behaviour (including sexual expression). Once the material conditions of disability changed, then social relations would follow, or so it was hoped.

This model of social being and social change drew heavily on earlier and contemporary identity social movements – around gender, race and sexual preference – though it was also heavily influenced by materialist (neo-Marxist) perspectives, which had argued that consciousness comes from practice in the world. In this sense disability politics had to recognise that disabled people needed to engage with the world, and demand the opportunity to be part of the wider scene. Escaping the ghetto was thus a paramount goal – given expression through a sea-change in disability policies from the early 1970s. The 'de-institutionalisation' trickle responded to the demand for social inclusion, and soon became a flood.

In this process of transformation, it became clearer that a culture of disability was possible – and indeed its shape began to emerge. Wider theories of social and cultural change, embodied in the various approaches to feminism and in the rapidly developing field of cultural studies, drew more attention to the cultural locations of people with disabilities, as in the work of Mairian Corker (Corker 1998 and this volume). Culture was mobilised within the realm of the new social movements of disability.

Disability as a cultural movement

The disability movement really began to emerge through a process of ideological and organisational change – the closure of large-scale residential institutions and the policy goal of full community integration. From the outset the integration goal was undermined by declining financial resources – few societies could reduce taxes (as most Western societies began to do from the late 1970s under the influence of new right market rationality) and support the high quality, intensive programs required by the new policies. The disjunction between the ideology of inclusion and rights, and the reality of homelessness, isolation and exclusion, focused the attention of many disability activists on the relation between theory and practice. The deepening awareness of the issues found political expression initially in the global UN Year of the Disabled Person (1981), then in the growing international NGO arguments for changes to the WHO definitions of disability, and then in the campaign for an international convention on the rights of people with disabilities. By the end of the twentieth century the claims of the disability movement reflected both the desire for cultural recognition and the demands for economic and social rights. One of the significant dimensions was the acceptance of 'sign' as a language, and the growing awareness this reflected of the cultural diversity of disability experiences.

While disability has not often been accorded the same ontological status as 'gender' or 'ethnicity', it is also clear that disability is as socially created and culturally expressed, as are gender and ethnicity. Disability as a status could be applied to people because of impairments which were congenital – genetic or the consequence of pre-birth exposure to dangerous substances (usually industrial or military); or acquired – through disease, through industrial injuries, or military wounds, or through accidents (often motor vehicle); or impairments could be produced through the declining capacities of the body and mind brought on by age or other diseases. In all such situations, social interventions could either prevent or ameliorate the consequences of the disability – they could either recognise the fundamental right of all members of society to equal participation, or they could consign disabled people to the margins and deny their right to active involvement in the social world.

The affirmation of identities of difference has been a characteristic of many social movements. The difficulty facing the disability movement has been gaining some purchase on the understanding that disability identity can play a positive and creative role in increasing the wider societal understanding of the human condition. The creation of positive identities of cultural difference for ethnic, racial or sexual minorities within larger societies has not always been easy – but it has been effective in recognising their moral worth. On the other hand, the wider society has become sensitised to disability as 'the difficulty, for both blind and sighted persons, lies in conceiving blindness as having something to say in a world understood as sighted' (Michalko 1998, p. 127). Singer (1999) has also pointed out the issues raised for the wider world by the hyper-sensitivities of Asperger's Syndrome people, with their 'nerd'-like capacities in relation to new computer technologies, and their capacities to read emotions, yet their difficulties in operating in live group interactions.

One way in which European societies have managed questions of rights and social justice has been through the creation of legislation banning discrimination against groups defined in terms of some socially important characteristic – such as gender or the much more controversial concept of 'race'. Discrimination on the grounds of race was outlawed in Western societies (though did not stop) in the years from about 1965 to 1980 – followed by prohibitions on gender grounds (usually meaning discrimination against women). However action on disability has only occurred in the last decade of the century, with landmark legislation in the USA in 1990, in Australia in 1992, and in the UK in 1999.

One feels that some disabled people portray their experiences as living in the world in which they are on temporary visas, never knowing when their condition may worsen or the society may withdraw crucial facilities required for survival. Their common experiences can be summarised as Robert Murphy does – 'as liminal people, the disabled confront each other as whole individuals, unseparated by social distinctions' (Murphy 1987, p. 134). The body and its 'troubles' move more centrally into individual consciousness, while identity becomes a more complex mesh of individual and social perceptions and responses. As part of the working through of these issues and the building of movements for social justice, disability activists speak of 'disability culture', a stratum of meaning and understanding that crosses disability types and conveys their shared sense of daunting challenges and profound insights.

Many disabled people experience being the object of inspection, pity, awe, dread or whatever – their presence is always noticed, or manifestly not noticed. When they enter the spaces of the abled Other, they know they will be seen as Other and different. In an important sense, then, disability culture seeks to re-valorise disability experiences, and turn upside down the devaluation that society normally accords them. These individually shared experiences, rendered into social questions through social contact between disabled people, form the bases for the development of a disability culture. This disability culture has been 'grown' by the movement, as a means of self-affirmation, solidarity and personal autonomy. The politics of identity have been as important a part of the disability movement as they have been of other oppressed groups seeking to recover their histories of separation and dispersal. Removal or rejection from family and home, and the search for roots and meaning has created for disability its own diaspora. In rebuilding identity the movement has begun to generate its own cultural institutions.

Some examples of the emerging cultural institutions of disability can be seen in the arts. Film festivals which feature films by and about disabled people, also provide a milieu to critique the 'mainstream', both for its parody and stereotyping of disability, and for its dual messages (to disabled and non-disabled people). Media awards are given by disability bodies to applaud good practice and indicate how disability need not be a negative social relationship. Furthermore disability culture affirms different embodiments through literature, drama, sport and music, to name but a few dimensions of cultural expression that can often bridge ethnic and national boundaries. UNESCO in conjunction with the Japan Broadcasting Corporation (NHK) sponsored a major travelling international exhibition of the arts – 'One heart, One world' – a compilation of 100 poems and 100 works of art by disabled artists from six countries.

Disability has its own cultural history, not just the cultural perceptions of disability by the wider society. It has its internal narratives, its own meanings, and its own yet-to-be-unearthed histories. Disability culture is evolving a sense of common originating moments (not of the individual's disability but of the calling-into-being of a community), a set of rituals and practices, and even a sense of an imaginary homeland, where disability is not the object of prejudice and oppression. The writing of disability histories plays a crucial role in the evolution of the sense of community, as does the inter-weaving of disability narratives into the whole history of a society in all its diversity (Longmore and Umansky 2001). The new ethnography of disability also extends and deepens the culture of the community, as in the work of Robert Murphy (1987) whose anthropological reflections on his own odyssey with disability reveal the value of ethnographic perspectives; and through the narrative ethnography of Gelya Frank (2000) in her account of the life of Diane DeVries.

The development of this wide-ranging disability culture has occurred through conflict with entrenched structures of cultural power that in the past have excluded or denied disabled participation. The stories have had to be rewritten, the truths torn from the suppressed experiences of disabled people. As cultural minorities have had to build their own histories and rediscover the strength of their own cultures, so too disability culture has been forged in interaction between diverse disabled people.

In summary, disability studies and the disability movement stress the crucial embodied aspect of all social relations – and that the deeply embedded assumptions about bodily normalcy which infuse most social theory have to be exposed for the contingent and tentative states they represent. How then do disability and multiculturalism engage – and what can be learnt from a deeper engagement?

● Crossover – disability, multiculturalism and reconciliation

The often universalistic logic of gender and race begin to unwind when they are tested by disabled people. Feminist theory has had to refashion its conception of the female body and the nature of identity under the trenchant criticisms from theorists such as Rosemary Garland Thomson (1997) and Carol Thomas (1999). Issues of desire, sexuality, reproductive rights, aesthetics, sexual choice, and the nature of families, have all been explored by disabled women committed to claiming spaces for women of difference – in bodily capacity, neurological orientation and health status (Meekosha 1998). Some feminists stress that the contemporary cosmopolitan fetishisation of traditional cultures can sustain enormous injustices towards women from ethnic communities through the reinforcement of misogynist patriarchal practices (Cohen and Howard 1999; Pettman 1996).

In recent years disabled people in Australia have raised similar concerns about both the multicultural movement and the Indigenous movement. The National Ethnic Disability Alliance has noted that the Australian Human Rights and Equal Opportunity Act allows the Immigration Department legally to exclude people with disabilities from coming to Australia, by emphasising their disabilities, and downplaying any consideration of their abilities. In the wider community, few mainstream disability services have been able to cope with cultural differences among their clients, so that ethnic minorities often receive the poorest services and the least attention. In the disability arena cultural values can become extremely contentious questions, as practitioners range in their responses from being overly solicitous of parental and family concerns (thus limiting client autonomy), through to a complete disregard for familial concerns as evidence of pre-modern superstition. Little expertise has been built in either the multicultural industry or the disability services area to develop effective programs.

The Indigenous situation is more complex again. Certain types of disability are widespread, if sometimes unrecognised as such, within Indigenous communities, as a consequence of the long colonial experience. Poorer levels of general health, blindness from glaucoma and diabetes, and developmental disabilities, contribute to the general social problems of the communities, as do increasingly dangerous acts by young men, showing up as motor vehicle accident injuries. Yet the social processes that disable Indigenous people are rarely identified by disability services as a matter of concern for policy. In part the National Indigenous Disability Network was created to raise awareness of these issues, and build more effective prevention, support and rights strategies.

At the crossover point, activist organisations have to face two problematic organisational environments: the disability world with its low level of awareness of and capacity to respond to cultural diversity, and the race and ethnic worlds with their political priorities that rarely locate disability as an issue at all. The intellectual challenges are as acute as those in practical politics. Each of these discourses contains its own legitimating structures in relation to authenticity, legitimacy, recognition and identity. These structures seem to echo Derrida's concept of *différence* – where they each act as the subterranean opponent of the other (Wolf 1994), destabilising the claims to categorical explanation.

As states are principally concerned about the relation between defined populations and defined territories, and expend significant resources asserting their definitions of both, control of the body and control of bodies sit very closely together. Population and citizenship policy marks the point of sharpest intersection, where population numbers, health, population sources and cultural acceptability all influence government action. Population policy has an external (immigration) and an internal (disability and health) dimension, though these areas may have rather different priorities. Thus in the 2001 Australian census, there were questions about language, country of birth, religion and heritage (identity). There was no question about disability – though Internet use was canvassed. Immigration policy has a long eugenicist prologue, with close connections made between physical appearance, cultural capital and moral hygiene. Similarly, disability policy still has strong eugenicist components, with the sterilisation of women with developmental and other disabilities regularly undertaken as a 'medical' procedure.

Population and the popular: disability engages with multiculturalism

The nation-building project contains many elements, though three are of particular importance here: the definition of citizenship and strategies for disciplining citizens; the conceptualisation of the nation and thereby those populations which have a legitimate role in nation building and agenda setting; and building of cultural identities. It is not often that governments stimulate public debate about these dimensions of the nation, but in early 2000 the Australian Citizenship Council issued its careful exploration of the meaning of Australian citizenship. It arrived at a set of seven core values it believed all Australians could commit to, without alienating anyone (Australian Citizenship Council 2000). The Citizenship Council reported to the Minister for Immigration and Multiculturalism. It is indicative of the conceptual and discursive boundaries between multiculturalism and disability (and indeed between disabled people and 'all Australians'), that there was no mention anywhere in the report of the citizenship issues affecting people with disabilities.

Yet the report talks much of Australian multiculturalism, and suggests it is a sufficiently encompassing phrase to allow all Australians to feel comfortable with it. So is the disability culture described above one of the cultures in multiculturalism (Peters 2000)? Whether we answer in the affirmative or not, important questions are raised. If yes, how should multicultural policies recognise disability culture; if not, how should governments ensure that the issues raised within disability culture receive a real and responsive airing? These questions can only be avoided by denying the possibility of the idea of a disability culture.

The Deaf community has become the sharpest focus for the discussion about what disability cultures might involve. The Deaf community has most adamantly advocated a cultural identity. Indeed the Deaf community sometimes rejects the label of disability altogether, claiming in the US context that American Sign is a language, and the Deaf have a culture as legitimate and potent as any immigrant or indigenous one. Furthermore, Deaf community activist Lois Bragg has argued that of disabled people only the Deaf could be a community, because the other disability sectors lack crucial dimensions of culture – a common language, a cohesive social community, a shared history, political solidarity and so forth (quoted in Peters 2000). Susan Peters' critique and many others – e.g. Pfeiffer's advocacy of disability culture as part of multiculturalism (Pfeiffer 1998) – reject such a narrow view, proposing rather that disability as a shared experience of a disabling society in fact does provide many of the conditions under which a shared culture is emerging. In part this may be formed in sub-cultures of particular impairments; it is also forged in the development of creative lifestyle alternatives to the submissive acceptance of oppression (Fleischer and Zames 2001).

The debate over the various meanings of multiculturalism will ensnare popular demagogues and scholars for a long time to come. Here we will propose that multiculturalism and its adjectival form 'multicultural' refer to two related phenomena: a) societies and smaller organisations which contain a variety of self-identifying groups whose internal self-definition depends on a communal narrative of shared experience (whether this is in a distinctive language etc.); and b) state policies which recognise this difference and seek to manage it (by recognition, denial, suppression, separation or whatever). Multiculturalism in the Australian context has emerged from a tumultuous series of arguments and political struggles over the nature of Australian society. Currently it tends to be used in the vernacular (and in much academic writing) to refer only to group relations which are predicated on 'ethnic' cultural differences. It does not usually refer to Indigenous cultures, which have other material claims against the notion that multiculturalism does not seek to address. It also usually excludes gay and lesbian culture, and as we have seen, does not involve itself at all with cultures of disability.

Disability studies can help open up these issues by exploring what embodiment means in each of the three critical areas: citizenship; nation building and cultural identity (Meekosha and Dowse 1997). In a complex democratic society, citizenship involves not only participation in formal political activities, but also a wider sense of responsibility for the mutual well-being of the community. Reciprocity, mutual aid, and communal action characterise democratic citizenship. This widespread definition indicates that the provision of social facilities needs to respect cultural differences, including those generated from struggles around recognition of the legitimacy of different lifestyles occasioned by impairments. But such respect of difference can only come from mutual recognition, and strategies of active citizenship open to all. To become active citizens also requires access to resources: thus a politics of recognition implies a politics of distribution. Active citizenship has to take account of different embodiments and how the practice of citizenship needs to be adjusted to ensure respect is realistically expressed.

The nation-building agenda has undergone serious critiques over the past few years, in particular concerning the idea that a 'mainstream' can dictate the total agenda and that special interests should be marginalised. In the practical policy arenas of disability 'reform', the Australian government has moved to demobilise disability groups (as it has done previously with ethnic and multicultural organisations). It proposed in 2000 to reduce the range of disability policy advice groups, and reintroduce distinctions on the basis of the medical model of disability. Furthermore peak bodies concerned with ethnic, gender and indigenous issues are under constant review and threat of closure, and the 'mainstream' medically defined groups – containing service providers and consumers – are to take on these responsibilities. Meanwhile, the struggles for disability rights which have taken place over the past twenty years are to be blocked, with 'mutual obligation' (the punitive device already used to reduce access in areas of unemployment benefit) being extended to people with impairments, although the activity test has not been imposed on them (McClure 2000). A significant number of these people are injured immigrant industrial workers, with little if any chance of re-employment, and for whom the requirements for job interviews and job seeking would be impossible to meet.

The exclusion of people with impairments from the nation-building process (joining in limbo non-Anglo immigrants, asylum seekers and Indigenous people) suggests that one crucial dimension of national solidarity – compassion – has been abandoned by the central government. The compassionate orientation that was evident in Australian social justice policies after 1983, has been replaced by a more vicious and hectoring tone, in which victims are urged to escape their situations and thus relieve the 'mainstream' of its responsibilities. Disability culture, by challenging the nation-building process to include the desires and sensibilities of people currently disabled by the nation, points to the way in which nation-building could become rather more inclusive across the board.

Multiculturalism has also become the terrain for debates on cultural identity – presenting analyses of post-colonial societies such as Australia where superordinate and subaltern relations are played out in terms of individual and group identities. In the post-modern globalising world identities are far more contingent, complex and fluid, undergoing change as the individual or group changes its place of residence or location for economic and social intersection. Class and gender are understood to cross-cut ethnic identities, producing a smear across the planet that decomposes into multitudes of ethno-scapes, each in constant change. Simple cultural prescriptions dissolve to be replaced by momentary arrangements; cultures feed into each other, producing *mélanges* with locality, sexuality, gender, class and disability strata. Disability activists swap notes on struggles and campaigns in Japan, Thailand, England and Australia. Bombay computer programmers buy homes in Palo Alto, living out their dream of California. Kosovars move restlessly across the world, seeking refuge wherever they can. Afghani women, those who manage to escape the oppression of the Taliban, are exposed to sexual assault and poverty, at the mercy of people smugglers in their flight towards refuge in countries resistant to their plight. Iranian writers pace the cages of concentration camps in the middle of Australian deserts.

All these people have bodies. Some refugees, their legs left as stumps from land mines, may find that Australia rejects them as 'disabled', whatever their capacities, splitting families. They discover that their state of defencelessness magnifies their vulnerability. Industrial workers, ageing and alone after forty years at the steelworks in Wollongong, eke out their lives in pain and isolation, in communities unable to speak their names or understand their cries. Immigrant women, hands bent with arthritis and wrists slashed to relieve the carpal pain caused by repetition strain injury, find themselves without sources of income after years on home sewing machines as clothing outworkers. Near the factory chimneys, children of immigrant parents grow up poisoned by lead, or their lungs heaving with asthmatic attacks.

What multicultural theory needs to understand is that industrial capitalism and the immigration process consume not just labour power but the bodies that deliver it. The experiences of disability have produced cultures which are as important in the lives of their bearers as ethnic or Indigenous experiences may be (indeed such separations are coarse and misdirected). Disability theory needs to understand the complex and subtle ways in which non-Anglo cultures interpret and offer support for people who come from different places and mobilise different world views.

Conclusion

The human rights issues revealed by the critical intersection of disability and multiculturalism as discourses of difference suggest that current theory in each case cannot account for the other. Thus despite a growing commonality in the political and social treatment by governments of unwanted and marginalised bodies, the social movements and the theoretical discussions that focus on ethnic or disability communities have yet to address the points of intersection and interaction.

When these theoretical realms meet with a shock of mutual recognition, we will see a greatly invigorated analytic and political project able to emerge. This project will reflect human rights to cultural expression and vital community life. It needs both a politics of recognition and a politics of redistribution, which validate the presence in the world of people with differing and perhaps contentious cultures, and also those whose being in the world does not fit the stereotypes of normality. The politics of difference are always embodied.

References

Australian Citizenship Council (2000) *For a New Australian Citizenship Century*, A.G.P.S., Canberra.

Barnes, C., Mercer, G. *et al.* (1999) *Exploring Disability: A Sociological Introduction*, Polity Press, Cambridge.

Barton, L. (1993) 'The Struggle for Citizenship: The case of disabled people', *Disability Handicap & Society* 8(3), pp. 235–248.

Barton, L. (1994) 'Disability, difference and the politics of definition', *Australian Disability Review*, 3, pp. 8–22.

Brace, M. (2000) 'UN Censures Treatment of Aborigines', *Guardian Weekly*.

Cohen, J. and Howard, M. (eds) (1999) *Is Multiculturalism Bad for Women?*, Princeton University Press, Princeton.

Corker, M. (1998) *Deaf and Disabled or Deafness Disabled*, Open University Press, Buckingham.

Disability Council of New South Wales (2000) *Inquiry into the Factors Responsible for the Increase in Prisoner Population*, Disability Council of New South Wales.

Finkelstein, V. (1988) 'To deny or not to deny disability', *Spinet*, 1(3), pp. 18–19.

Fleischer, D.Z. and Zames, F. (2001) *The Disability Rights Movement*, Temple University Press, Philadelphia.

Foucault, M. (1994) *Ethics – subjectivity and truth*, Allen Lane, London.

Frank, G. (2000) *Venus on Wheels*, UCP, Berkeley.

Fraser, N. (1995) 'From Redistribution to Recognition? Dilemmas of Justice in a "Post-Socialist" Age', *New Left Review*, 212, pp. 68–93.

Gilson, S. and Depoy, E. (2000) 'Multiculturalism and disability: a critical perspective', *Disability and Society*, **15**(2).

Honneth, A. (1995) *The Struggle for Recognition: The Moral Grammar of Social Conflicts*, Polity, Cambridge.

Longmore, P. and Umansky, L. (eds) (2001) *The New Disability History*, New York University Press, New York.

McClure, P. (2000) *Participation Support for a More Equitable Society – Final report of the Reference Group on Welfare Reform*, Department of Family and Community Services, Canberra.

McLaren, P. (1994) 'White terror and oppositional agency: towards a critical multiculturalism' in Goldberg, D., *Multiculturalism: a critical reader*, Blackwell, Cambridge, MA, pp. 45–74.

Meekosha, H. (1998) 'Body Battles: Bodies, Gender and Disability' in Shakespeare, T., *The Disability Reader: Social Science Perspectives*, Cassell, London.

Meekosha, H. and Dowse, L. (1997) 'Enabling Citizenship: Gender, Disability and Citizenship', *Feminist Review*, (Autumn), pp. 49–72.

Michalko, R. (1998) *The Mystery of the Eye and the Shadow of Blindness*, University of Toronto Press, Toronto.

Murphy, R. (1987) *The Body Silent*, Henry Holt & Co., New York.

Nirje, B. (1985) 'The Basis and Logic of the Normalization Principle', *Australia and New Zealand Journal of Developmental Disabilities*, **11**(2), pp. 65–68.

Oliver, M. (1996) *Understanding Disability*, Macmillan, London.

Pernick, M. (1997) 'Defining the Defective: Eugenics, Aesthetics, and Mass Culture in Early-Twentieth Century America', in Mitchell, D. and Snyder, S., *The Body and Physical Difference: Discourses of disability*, Michigan, University of Michigan Press, pp. 89–110.

Peters, S. (2000) 'Is There a Disability Culture? A Syncretisation of Three Possible World Views', *Disability and Society*, **15**(4), pp. 583–601.

Pettman, J. (1996) *Worlding Women: A feminist international politics*, Allen and Unwin, Sydney.

Pfeiffer, D. (1998) 'An Essay on Multiculturalism and Sadness', *Disability Studies Quarterly*, **18**(1), pp. 27–29.

Rozen, S. (1999) *Liebe Perla*. Israel/Germany, film produced by Edna Kowarsky.

Singer, J. (1999) 'Why can't you be normal for once in your life?' From a "problem with no name" to the emergence of a new category of difference', in Corker, M. and French, S., *Disability Discourse*, Open University Press, Buckingham, pp. 59–67.

Taylor, C. (1994) 'The Politics of Recognition' in Guttman, A., *Multiculturalism*, Princeton University Press, Princeton NJ, pp. 25–73.

Thomas, C. (1999) *Female Forms: Experiencing and understanding disability*, Open University Press, Buckingham.

Thomson, R. (1997) *Extraordinary Bodies: Figuring Physical Disability In American Culture and Literature*, Columbia University Press, New York.

Williams, Hon. Daryl (2001) Answer to Question on Notice, 9th Attorney-General's NGO Forum on Domestic Human Rights, Canberra, Commonwealth of Australia, Department of Attorney-General, 19 April.

Wolf, S. (1994) 'Comment' in Gutmann, A., *Multiculturalism: Examining the politics of recognition*, Princeton University Press, Princeton, pp. 75–85.

Wolfensberger, W. (1983) 'Social Role Valorization: A Proposed New Term for the Principle of Normalization', *Mental Retardation*, **21**(6), pp. 234–239.

Young, I.M. (1997) 'Unruly Categories: A Critique of Nancy Fraser's Dual Systems Theory', *New Left Review*, **222**, pp. 147–160.

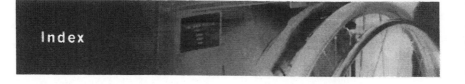